These books have  Strong Start Team working in partnership with Milk and You.

Strong Start are qualified Early Years professionals commissioned by Public Health to provide the universal part of the Children's Centre Services offer for West and North Northants
strongstartteam@westnorthants.gov.uk
07880136070

Milk&You are Public Health commissioned breast feeding peer support volunteers trained to offer guidance on infant feeding.
07949353423

Str9ng Start

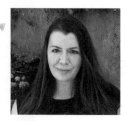

About the author

Professor Amy Brown is based in the Department of Public Health, Policy and Social Sciences at Swansea University in the UK where she leads the MSc in Child Public Health. With a background in psychology, she first became interested in the many barriers women face when breastfeeding after having her first baby. Three babies and a PhD later she has spent the last twelve years exploring psychological, cultural and societal barriers to breastfeeding, with an emphasis on understanding how we can better support women to breastfeed and subsequently raise breastfeeding rates. Her primary focus is how we can shift our perception of breastfeeding as an individual mothering issue, to a wider public health responsibility, with consideration how we can make societal changes to protect and encourage breastfeeding.

Professor Brown has published over 60 papers exploring the barriers women face in feeding their baby during the first year. In 2016 she published her first book *Breastfeeding Uncovered: Who really decides how we feed our babies*, followed by *Why Starting Solids Matters* in 2017 and *The Positive Breastfeeding Book* in 2018. She is a regular Huffington Post blogger, aiming to change the way we think about breastfeeding, mothering and caring for our babies.

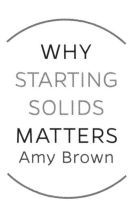

WHY
STARTING
SOLIDS
MATTERS
Amy Brown

Why Starting Solids Matters (Pinter & Martin Why It Matters 8)

First published by Pinter & Martin Ltd 2017, reprinted 2019

©2017 Amy Brown

ISBN 978-1-78066-500-9

Also available as an ebook

Pinter & Martin Why It Matters ISSN 2056-8657
Series editor: Susan Last
Index: Helen Bilton
Design: Rebecca Longworth
Cover Design: Blok Graphic, London
Cover illustration: Donna Smith
Proofreader: Sarah Dronfield

British Library Cataloguing-in-Publication Data

A catalogue record for this book is available from the British Library.

Set in Minion

Printed and bound in the EU by Hussar

This book has been printed on paper that is sourced and harvested from sustainable forests and is FSC accredited.

Pinter & Martin Ltd
6 Effra Parade
London SW2 1PS

pinterandmartin.com

Contents

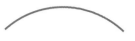

Introduction

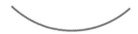

I started writing this book a few days after Christmas. Flicking through social media, among photos of smiling babies chewing wrapping paper and toddlers preferring the box to their actual toys, I noticed a theme in parents' comments.

'My mother said he should be sleeping through the night by now and I need to give him something more.'

'My sister said her baby is on three meals a day already and he's a month younger than mine.'

'My granny said they gave solids by six weeks when her babies were little.'

Most of these comments came from parents who had a baby four or five months old – below the age at which the World Health Organization recommends solids are first introduced.

A note about terminology

In this book I use the term 'starting solids' in preference to 'weaning'. The term 'weaning' can be confusing, because in some countries, and in some scientific papers, 'weaning' means the end of breastfeeding, rather than the introduction of complementary foods alongside breast or formula feeding. In the UK many people use 'weaning' to mean starting solids (as in 'baby-led weaning', which is discussed throughout the book). 'Starting solids' avoids any confusion: I am talking about introducing complementary foods alongside continued milk feeding.

How and when babies are introduced to solid foods is something many new parents worry about. Just when you've seemingly got to grips with milk feeding, someone asks when you're going to start giving them solids, and how you're going to do it… and it can feel like a very loaded question. Many parents haven't thought about it before their baby arrives, but the newborn weeks pass quickly and it won't be long before you're asked about your plans. I can remember having a conversation about feeding with my health visitor when my oldest child was a little baby. I planned to breastfeed. For exactly six months. As that was what the guidelines said.

'And then…?' she gently asked.

I was stumped. No idea. You just got on with it and gave them solids at six months didn't you? But when I started to think about it, it suddenly seemed a lot more complicated. Why six months? How much? When? What foods? Why? Do I need to still give milk feeds? What about vitamin drops? Does it matter if I spoon feed? What if they don't like it? And this was before anyone else chimed in. When parents are struggling with sleep deprivation and a tremendous sense of responsibility for keeping a small thing alive, the whole question of starting solids seems overwhelming.

And then there's the emotional element. Starting solids may not be as hot a topic as decisions about breast or formula feeding, but it's certainly debated by family, friends and the good folk of the internet. Those around you often have strong opinions, and the 'rules' have likely changed since your parents were introducing solid foods to you. Food, after all, is not just about nutrition, and feeding babies often gets entangled with notions of love, care, culture and more. Who to listen to? And where to find good evidence-based information? How do you know what's genuinely helpful, and not simply trying to make money out of your desire to do the best for your baby?

In the developed world we are lucky to have safe, nutritious food options and vitamin drops as a safety net. Introducing solid foods safely and sufficiently matters, but it is not generally a dangerous time, as it is for many babies in poorer areas of the world. The World Health Organization describes how malnutrition has been responsible, directly or indirectly, for around 7 million deaths annually among children under five in developing countries. Over two-thirds of those deaths occur during the first year of life.

In more privileged contexts, parents also worry about introducing solid foods and have many questions and concerns. This is normal and reasonable: good nutrition is important for our health throughout our lives. But how much do we really need to worry? To put it in very simple terms, introducing solids is about moving your baby gradually from an entirely milk diet to one that includes a range of family foods by around 12 months. Despite grave warnings from some about 'deficiencies', it's not about diving in at the deep end with three meals a day, or breast or formula milk suddenly losing its nutrition, Cinderella-style, at the stroke of midnight on the day your baby turns six months old. Think of it more as a gradual learning experience – your baby will learn how to handle foods, what they taste and feel like, how to chew and swallow, and become part of your family's experience of eating.

The phrase 'food before one is just for fun' is bandied about online, particularly on US websites and forums, to describe the process of introducing solid foods. There is a lot of sense in this, but it can be interpreted in the wrong way. I think a better version might be 'food before one is *mainly* for fun'. Breast or formula milk remains an important and nutritious part of your baby's diet until they are one (and beyond). The transition from a milk-only diet to one that includes solids should certainly be gradual. There is no need to rush, and as we will see in later chapters, at first babies will only need a small proportion of their calories from solids (about 20–25%). This gradually increases as the months pass. Milk is still an important source of energy and nutrients in the second year of life, and breastfeeding is encouraged to age two and beyond.

However, babies are born with stores of minerals (particularly iron), which are not present in high levels in milk. These are gradually used up during the period of exclusive milk feeding. They therefore need to start getting them from a variety of foods by around six months. They don't need large amounts, and the need to ensure that they get these minerals doesn't mean the process of introducing foods can't be fun.

Offering a wide variety of foods to your baby will help them to get a good range of nutrients. Tastes and textures are important too – it must be strange to go from only drinking milk (although the taste of breastmilk does change slightly according to what the mother has eaten), to consuming foods that taste, feel and smell different, and learning to chew and swallow and not spit things back out. We needn't over-complicate the process or agonise over it – as we will see. But making sense of the seemingly conflicting, biased or partial information parents are given about introducing foods can be challenging. This is partly due to political, economic and commercial influences, and I will explore this in more detail. Always consider where information has come from and what the authors stand to gain financially. (Yes, I am looking at you formula companies and your suspicious sponsorship of way too much stuff in this area.) As the World Health Organization emphasises:

> *'Mothers, fathers and other caregivers should have access to objective, consistent and complete information about appropriate feeding practices, free from commercial influence.'*

This brings me to the aim of this book – to look at the guidance behind introducing solid foods, the evidence behind it, and the wider context. We'll look at what babies really need in terms of solid foods: when, how and why? How did we get to where we are now? Is there one right way to introduce solid foods, or is it better to respond to your individual baby's needs? (Spoiler – responsiveness is the key.)

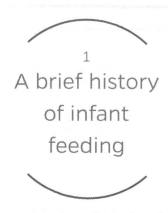

1

A brief history of infant feeding

To understand current influences on introducing solid foods, it's a good idea to start at the beginning and consider how our natural behaviour fits with what we do now. What did we do before baby cookbooks, the baby food industry and advertising? Anthropology has a lot to tell us about what the human body is naturally designed to do.

Of course, 'natural' does not always mean best. Natural can be deadly and many babies would have starved, died of infections or been malnourished before science, medicines and technology vastly improved our health. However, sometimes we forget what our bodies are designed to do. Our interventions may save the lives of the most vulnerable, but too much interference can have unintended consequences for the rest.

When you think of introducing solid foods to babies, what comes to mind? Family foods? Commercial products? 'How to' books, blenders and miniature plastic boxes? Mess? Always mess. Examining our first thoughts on the subject is interesting, because understanding where our ideas come from can help us think critically about why we believe certain things. Is our behaviour around introducing solid foods necessary? Or has it been influenced by social, economic and political factors?

Historians and anthropologists have investigated our eating practices over the centuries, including evidence of what foods babies were given and when. Skeletal examinations have helped us estimate how long babies were typically breastfed for and when other foods were introduced. Birth spacing is another useful tool – the longer the birth interval between babies, the more likely it is that they were breastfed for longer, with their mothers benefitting from the contraceptive effect of unrestricted breastfeeding. Further information has been obtained from philosophical and medical writing and artifacts, including instruments used to feed babies, drawings and notes.

Human beings, as mammals, are unique in their diet and feeding practices, not least because of our different development. While many mammals are born able to walk within a few hours of life, it takes us a year or longer to get to the same stage. This is mainly because we are busy still growing our brains – our heads would be too big to be born if we were born at the same stage of physical development as other mammals. This means that although other mammals will have their mothers' milk, many grazing animals, for example, will also be able to 'forage' on the food around them and feed themselves from very early on. This obviously varies considerably across mammalian groups, but as a species we are helpless for longer than many others. Even the most determined human baby takes several months to learn how to move around to find food. Socialisation means that we don't generally let babies just crawl off and eat what they want, in the way a horse might 'let' its foal graze. We have also developed the ability to modify and mix food sources in a way that other mammals cannot, meaning our potential diet is far more complex.

Our nutritional histories reflect this. It appears that babies were not typically introduced to solids until much later than they are now. Birth spacing data from the Palaeolithic era suggests that there were fairly long gaps between babies – at least two years and more like three, four or five. One reason for this is that until around 10,000 years ago taking milk from another species to give to babies was not really an option, so mothers breastfed until their children were old enough to forage and feed themselves. If they couldn't be breastfed, a wet nurse was found. If this couldn't happen a pap-type mixture of grains and water would be given. However, giving anything apart from breastmilk was risky and associated with high mortality rates – not only because of the lack of infection-fighting breastmilk, but because the replacement food did not provide adequate nutrition and may have been contaminated.[1]

Historical documents from Roman times suggest that although some babies were given milk and eggs before being weaned from the breast, fruit and vegetables were only given after breastfeeding was stopped. Religious documents such as the Bible and Talmud make references to this occurring at around 2–3 years old. Hippocrates – the ancient Greek physician credited with being the father of modern medicine – is thought to have believed that babies should be introduced to solid foods at around the time they got their first teeth, and records suggest that this was likely the case.

Physicians Soranus (circa 98BC–AD138) and Galen (circa AD130–200AD) gave specific dietary guidance for babies. Both believed that the first food should be honey (we now know that babies who have honey before 12 months are at increased risk – albeit small – of botulism). Soranus felt that solids should be introduced no earlier than 40 days, but preferably around six months, while Galen stuck with the idea of after the first tooth. First foods recommended by Soranus included cereal, bread, milk, porridge, eggs and… wine. Yes, wine. Galen suggested bread, vegetables, meat and milk, but didn't believe wine was such a good idea for babies. Weaning from the breast should be gradual and occur at around two years (Soranus) and three years (Galen).

Some years later Avicenna, a Persian physician (circa 980–1036), recommended that children be breastfed for as long as possible as *it is the most appropriate food for growth and development'*. He also believed honey should be the first food, but that introduction of solid foods should wait until the child requested it. Complementary foods should include pre-chewed bread, then normal bread, honey and milk… and wine (diluted!).

During the 16th and 17th century complementary foods were introduced at around 8–9 months (alongside breastfeeding for two or three years), but some started to introduce food earlier as wet-nursing began to decline. If a woman could not or did not want to breastfeed, instead of asking a wet nurse to breastfeed her child she might use foods instead. These were typically paps and bread sops consisting of a mixture of liquids (milk, vegetable or meat stock, beer or wine), cereals and additives such as sugar, herbs or spices. Sometimes eggs or meat were added. These were actually quite nutritionally sound, but over time the milk and animal stocks were replaced by water and the eggs and meat were no longer added. This meant that vitamins, calcium and iron were lacking, and illnesses such as scurvy and rickets became more common. Contamination of the utensils used to feed these foods also increased the risk of infections.[2]

As industrialisation meant that more women went to work in the growing cities, breastfeeding continued to decline. The advent of formula milks in the late 19th century encouraged the earlier introduction of solid foods. The 1911 edition of *Diseases of Infancy and Childhood* recommended that vegetables should be introduced after three years (once the child was weaned from the breast). However, by 1929 the same book was recommending giving solid foods, specifically cereals, at nine months, and most babies were having solids towards the end of the first year. Notably vegetables were still to be delayed, because there was a lot of suspicion around them. Many believed that they were responsible for diseases such as cholera, dysentery and fevers, especially among young children, and they were felt to add bulk rather than nutrients to a child's diet. It wasn't until later that vitamins and minerals and their benefits were 'discovered'.

A study conducted in 1933 by Cornell University found that the average age of introduction to solid foods was about seven and a half months, although foods such as meat and fish were introduced closer to one year. However, by the early 1950s it was recommended that babies were introduced to fruits and vegetables by four months of age. Just a decade later, in 1960, over 80% of babies had received some type of complementary food by *one month* of age. By 1970 many physicians suggested introducing foods at six weeks, although some 'delayed' until three months.[3]

Specific guidance for mothers

The change in timing of introduction to solid foods in the 1930s came hand-in-hand with more specific guidance and rules aimed at mothers, not just about timing of solid foods, but what foods should be given and when. Pediatricians became more involved, but so did self-appointed 'parenting experts', who developed strict ideas about complementary foods. For example, in 1929 the United States Children's Bureau published *Infant Care* guidance that had very specific rules around when foods should be introduced.

> '*When you give the baby his first taste of cereal you are offering him the first of a series of new experiences which he will eventually meet with satisfaction and enjoyment but which are as yet entirely unknown to him. Much of his future health, both physical and mental, depends on how you teach him to meet new experiences*'.

Specifically, the guidance stated that babies should be introduced to solid foods at around five to six months, although fruit juices were recommended from the first month of life in order to increase vitamin C intake and prevent scurvy. Babies should receive one teaspoonful twice a day of either orange or tomato juice, increasing to one tablespoon twice a day by the third month.

Babies were also to be given solid foods in a strict routine (matching the strict routines for milk feeding recommended at the time). They should be given cereals from five to six months, specifically at 10am and 6pm. In between they should have a mixture of egg yolk and vegetables mashed through a strainer. Egg yolks were recommended for their iron content and babies should have a whole egg yolk per day. Vegetables should be of the dark leafy variety for iron and vitamins A, B and C. Spinach was seen as the best vegetable (although we now know that despite its seemingly high iron content, the iron is very poorly absorbed). Cod liver oil should be given for vitamin D to prevent rickets. Stewed fruits could also be given to regulate the bowels. Potatoes should be delayed until 10 months in case babies developed a preference for them.

Overall complementary foods should equate to around 2–3 ounces of food per pound of body weight per day.[4]

The Depression of the 1930s and the Second World War brought lower incomes and food shortages, placing young children at a risk of undernourishment. However, advances in public health meant that the importance of infant nutrition and growth for longer-term health was recognised, and campaigns such as 'Doctor Carrot', emphasising the importance of vegetables and nutrients for young children and babies, and 'Don't let Dad get all the meat' were influential.[5] This continued to pave the way for more directive advice about how babies should be fed and a number of parenting experts published their own guidelines.

Truby King was a doctor who published a number of books on 'mothercraft' in the early half of the 20th century. These were very influential in New Zealand, Australia and the UK until around the 1940s. King was a supporter of breastfeeding (although he did have some strange ideas, recommending four-hourly feeds and no feeding at night) and recommended introducing solid foods no later than nine months. He advised that babies should be introduced to one solid food at a time – importantly by spoon, as many at the time were advising that foods should be added to bottles. Food should be mashed or finely sieved until two years of age, when harder foods such as raw apple could be introduced. Although Truby King was very much a believer in strict routines in terms of timings for milk and solid feeding, he did not recommend persuading the child to eat when they did not want to as he believed that *food tastes and habits are formed which may last a lifetime*.[6]

Not all parenting experts were so moderate. I think it is fair to say that Walter Sackette, a physician who published a book in 1953 called *Bringing up babies; a family doctor's practical approach to child care*, had very different views. Sackette believed in routines for babies, and that mothers should fit around the nursing staff when in hospital after giving birth. Newborn infants were only to have four milk feeds a day – precisely at 6am, 12pm, 6pm and 12am, as those times were *'the most workable ones in keeping with hospital routine'.* However, by three weeks he advised that the 12am feed should be dropped *'…having fully served its purpose, which was not to pacify the infant but his parents, grandparents, neighbours and doubting friends'.* Sackette's beliefs about introducing solid foods were even more remarkable. Sackette believed that if young babies could be given vitamin drops, they could have solid foods too. He recommended that babies be given cereals while they were still in the hospital (at 12 noon and 12 midnight as *'this is the handiest time for nurses in the hospital to get out on the floor and teach mothers how to give this cereal'*). He noted:

> *'don't be surprised to see baby eat his first cereal with gusto and a surprising dexterity … you needn't worry about the baby being able to handle the semi-solid cereal mixture. Research has shown that a baby's digestive tract will not be harmed by any food he can swallow'.*

Sackette never did elaborate on what research this was, but to those who questioned whether giving solids to babies who were only a few days old was a good idea he responded:

> *'I suspect that those authorities who claim that muscles for swallowing solid food are not properly developed until four months of age have made this idea up in their own minds and have never actually tried feeding solids to a newborn'.*

Sackette had a strict timetable for when foods should be given and in what order. The use of 'days' is not a typo.

- *2–3 days: cereal (oatmeal and barley)*
- *10 days: strained vegetables (peas, beans, carrots)*
- *17 days: strained fruits (applesauce, peaches, pears)*
- *3 weeks: orange juice*
- *4 weeks: strained meats*
- *5 weeks: custards*
- *6 weeks: soups*
- *7 weeks: mashed bananas*
- *8 weeks: egg*

Finally, by nine weeks baby could be offered *'bacon and eggs, just like Dad!... The saltiness and bacony taste is most acceptable to baby'*. While I agree that 'bacony' should definitely be a word, I do not think that giving babies salty food at two months old is sensible.[7]

Fortunately not everyone agreed with Sackette. In 1968 Dr Spock, author of one of the biggest-selling parenting manuals, who promoted the idea that mothers knew more than they thought they did, published his thoughts on solid foods. Spock was an advocate of allowing babies to self-feed as early as possible, believing in the importance of allowing them to explore the textures and tastes of food in their own time. His approach fits quite neatly with current recommendations by the World Health Organization to promote responsive feeding.

The birth of the baby foods market

The earlier introduction of solid foods, and specific ideas about what babies should be eating, went hand in hand with a move away from giving babies family foods, in favour of specially prepared infant foods. Arguably, the development of infant formula paved the way for other manufactured baby foods. 'Liebig's food', developed by Baron Justus Von Liebig in 1867, was the first infant formula, and was marketed as being virtually identical to mother's milk… at least in terms of containing protein, carbohydrate and fat. However, its ingredients were cows' milk, potassium bicarbonate and wheat and malt flours. These were then dried into a powder.

Similar products followed, some consisting of powdered milk to be mixed with water, while others were a supplement that you added to cows' milk. Henri Nestlé developed 'Nestlé's milk food', which was basically wheat rusks crumbled into sweet condensed milk, dried and sold as granules that could be mixed with milk or water. These products were followed by many similar grain mixtures that were something between milk and solid foods.[8]

Commercial complementary foods for babies did not really emerge onto the market until the late 1920s, when a number of social and economic factors came together to ensure that there was a ready market. The concept of infant food products had been introduced with infant formula, so mothers were primed to buy products specifically aimed at babies. Manufacturing advances meant that canned and packaged goods had come down in price. Alongside this there was a growing trust of science, medicine and products when it came to making health-related choices, and this included feeding babies. If a product was recommended by experts and had scientific claims attached, many people viewed it as superior to their normal family food.

It was also at around this time that scientists 'discovered' vitamins and minerals and realised that fruits and vegetables were the best sources. It was common to boil such foods extensively to rid them of feared diseases, compromising their nutritional value. In 1937 the American Medical Council declared that home-prepared foods could be used to feed babies: *'properly prepared, [they] are not inferior in nutritive value to the commercial product'*. The implication was clear: commercial products were better and more nutritious. The new baby food industry extolled the virtues of canned goods, which retained vitamins and minerals. Literacy rates, which had increased sharply, meant that more and more mothers were able to read the nutritional claims and information on goods, and the advertising used to persuade them the products were needed.

As the 20th century progressed, more and more women entered the workplace. The notion of 'time-saving' became very important as people tried to juggle work and family life. Using pre-prepared products and technological devices to save time and effort was seen as optimal.

Market conditions for commercial specialised baby foods were thus ideal. The first baby food is believed to have been sold by Clapp's Baby Foods, who developed 'baby soup' (essentially beef broth with added vegetables and cereal) in 1921. The promotional story went that Mrs Clapp was ill and unable to fully breastfeed her baby, so Mr Clapp valiantly stepped in and designed a baby food, which the child supposedly thrived on. The next step was obviously to sell this product to others – which he did fairly successfully, although what he really did was to pave the way for the biggest success story in infant food manufacturing in the USA – Gerber Foods.

Gerber were already manufacturing other canned goods. However in 1928 they launched a new baby food line, supposedly because Daniel Gerber's wife Dorothy was so tired of having to laboriously hand-strain vegetables for their seven-month-old daughter that she urged her husband to create something more convenient. Within a year the company had launched tins of special baby food including strained peas, prunes, carrots and spinach.

Although these foods were initially met with suspicion – why would canned foods be better for infants than home-made foods? – advertising and promotional campaigns aimed to convince mothers that these foods were needed. These included advertising in medical journals and ladies' magazines, and research to show that the foods were safe and maintained the vitamin content. Much was made of how convenient and time-saving the products were, while being supposedly far higher in vitamins and minerals than homemade foods. One physician was so taken by the idea that he conducted research on a small number of babies by introducing them to Gerber's strained vegetables at just six weeks old – he reported no negative side effects.

The campaigns had the desired effect and in 1930 Gerber sold 842,000 cans, rising to 1,311,500 in 1931 and 2,259,818 in 1932. These figures are impressive in themselves, but even more so against the economic backdrop of the Great Depression. Sales continued to grow, and during the Second World War the products were minimally rationed. By 1945 Gerber baby food products (the company had stopped making any other canned goods) turned over an estimated $100 million a year. By 1952 this figure had doubled.

Other baby food manufacturers of course sprang up. The USA led the way, but similar trends were seen in the UK, Europe and other Western countries. In the USA Gerber always held the biggest market share. As manufactured, specialised baby foods became more widely available, the perception that they were necessary, and at ever-earlier ages, also became more widespread. Fewer and fewer women were breastfeeding for any length of time.

The main baby food manufacturers positioned themselves as supportive and caring. Nestlé set up a 'department of advice for mothers' to support women introducing solids. Free coupons were sent out to 'help' with the expense. Gerber played the 'cute baby' card, choosing a pencil drawing of a rather young-looking baby as its iconic logo. Parents trusted the companies, seeing them as caring experts.[3]

By the 1970s the most common age of starting solid foods in the UK was at three or four weeks, with one study finding the youngest introduction at two days old.[9] Almost all babies were weaned onto solid foods by three months, and despite the Department of Health and Social Security (DHSS) advocating the delay of solid foods until after 4 months of age in 1974, bottle-fed babies were being weaned at an average age of 8.3 weeks and breastfed babies at 13.8 weeks in the late 1970s.[10]

However, this situation was not to last. Just as a number of factors had come together to cause the boom in the baby food industry, a number of factors were to transpire against it. Readily available contraception (and therefore choice for women) meant that the birth rate began to fall. Political thinking moved away from submitting to power, to opposing it. The increasing variety and availability of fresh foods meant that people were starting to cook again rather than use canned goods. Inflation meant that people wanted to save money, but technological advances meant that they could afford kitchen gadgets for their homes. More importantly, research was starting to focus on the impact of what we fed our babies. Although much research centred on examining the impact of breastmilk, the timing of solid foods was implicated. Research started to emerge that highlighted the benefits of delaying solid foods, rather than giving it as soon as possible.

Critics started to question the content of baby food. Although the main ingredient had to be listed, the quantities did not. This was a red flag to critics, who pointed out that dog food had to have specific nutritional information on the label.

Concerns were also raised about the addition of salt, added sugar and additives to baby food. Newspapers cottoned onto the fact that stories around issues like these could be used to shock the public (and sell papers).

In the USA these revelations led to a White Paper being published by medical doctors, public health officials and children's advocates, calling for action. Criticisms included the timing of introduction of baby foods, their composition and the lack of regulation of baby foods, as well as misleading advertising strategies. The paper was signed by 58 members of Congress, who together called for better advertising control and regulation.[3]

Finally, in 1981 the World Health Organization launched the International Code of Marketing of Breast-Milk Substitutes, which forbids companies from marketing breastmilk substitutes (and bottles and teats) for babies under six months old. This was primarily aimed at formula milk manufacturers, but many baby food manufacturers fell foul of its provisions too if they were marketing solid foods for infants under six months old. Manufacturers like Gerber, which was using an image of a baby that was clearly under six months old as a logo, were told under no uncertain terms to stop it. At least, they were in countries that put the provisions of the Code into their national law. Neither the US nor the UK has fully implemented the Code, even today.[11]

Early introduction of solids remained the norm, but in 1994 the recommendations were changed to say that solid foods should be introduced at four to six months. This meant that although in 1990 over 70% of mothers had introduced solid foods by three months (with only 6% waiting until after four months), by 2000 only 24% had introduced solids by three months. With a further change in recommendations to delay solids until around 6 months in 2001, by 2005 only 10%

had introduced by three months (and 51% by 4 months) and by 2010 it was just 5% (and 30% by four months).[12] The tide had turned.

What's clear from this brief survey of infant feeding is that throughout history babies have survived, and in many cases thrived, on a wide range of diets despite dubious advice and interference from self-styled experts and those interested in making money. What's also clear is that the knowledge we now have shows us that how babies are fed is important for both their short-term survival and their long-term health.

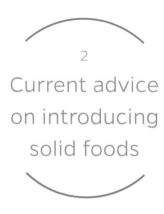

2

Current advice on introducing solid foods

Since 2001 the World Health Organization (WHO) has recommended that babies receive their first solid foods at around six months of age.[1] The majority of health organisations around the world have adopted these guidelines. Some of these are summarised below:

- UK Department of Health: *'Breastmilk is the best form of nutrition for infants. Exclusive breastfeeding is recommended for the first six months (26 weeks) of an infant's life. Six months is the recommended age for the introduction of solid foods for infants. Breastfeeding (and/or breastmilk substitutes, if used) should continue beyond the first six months, along with appropriate types and amounts of solid foods'.*[2]
- American Academy of Pediatrics: *'Babies should be exclusively breastfed for about the first six months of life. This means your baby needs no additional foods (except Vitamin D) or fluids unless medically indicated.*

> *Babies should continue to breastfeed for a year and for as long as is mutually desired by the mother and baby. Breastfeeding should be supported by your physician for as long as it is the right choice for you and your baby. Solid foods need to be introduced to ensure that your baby gets proper nutrition around six months of age.*[3]

- European Society for Paediatric Gastroenterology Hepatology and Nutrition (ESPGHAN): *'Exclusive or full breast-feeding for about six months is a desirable goal. Complementary feeding (i.e. solid foods and liquids other than breastmilk or infant formula and follow-on formula) should not be introduced before 17 weeks and not later than 26 weeks.'*[4]
- Australian Department of Health: *'Breastfeeding provides babies with the best start in life and is a key contributor to infant health. Australia's dietary guidelines recommend exclusive breastfeeding of infants until six months of age, with the introduction of solid foods at around six months and continued breastfeeding until the age of 12 months – and beyond, if both mother and infant wish'.*[5]

Why six months? What's the evidence?

In the previous chapter we looked at how recommendations about the timing of introduction to solid foods have changed over the years. They have now been at six months for 16 years. You may hear it suggested that the guidelines 'keep changing all the time', but really, they don't. There have been just two changes in the last 23 years (in 1994 and 2001).

However, it sometimes seems that the timing of introduction of solids is one of the most fiercely debated topics in nutrition and baby care literature. There are hundreds – if not thousands – of research articles discussing the issue. Some argue strongly for six months, others suggest earlier introduction, some are inconclusive. This is always going to be the case with human research – unless you literally 'breed' genetically identical babies and keep them in sterile laboratories with identical experiences, you're never going to exactly know. (That sort of experiment is of course completely unethical.)

What really matter are the *patterns* in research – if we weigh up the studies, which way do the scales fall? Pathways are important too – these suggest possible explanations for the findings. How might our internal and external physiological development give hints to when solids might best be introduced? Anthropology and child development really come into their own here. If a randomised controlled trial shows a benefit of waiting until six months, is that actually plausible? Does six months make sense in terms of babies' natural ability? When would babies naturally self-feed? What do other mammals do? When did we introduce solids in history?

And of course then there are the politics. Baby food is deeply entwined in social experience, economic factors and politics. We saw earlier that industry has affected the timing of introduction of solid foods, and, as we will see later when we look at homemade versus commercial foods, it continues to have a strong influence. Unfortunately industry tends to have far more money and power to put behind research than governments, as it stands to make a profit from the outcomes. Good health doesn't make a profit directly in the same way – although we know it does eventually in terms of improved population health. Thus much of the research on baby food is funded by baby food manufacturers – which makes it difficult to trust the findings. If a baby food company produces research concluding that you should introduce solids at three months rather than six (thus buying their product for an additional three months), is it really trustworthy? Remember too that when research is funded by industry, this may lead to publication bias. Don't like the findings? Don't publish.

Research that tackles the issue of timing of solid foods tends to focus on two key elements: when should solids be introduced, and the duration of exclusive breastfeeding. The two are obviously linked – introducing solids means an end to exclusive breastfeeding – but together these two elements help us understand the pathways of effect. Is it the introduction of solids that matters? Or the reduction in – or cessation of – breastfeeding? What happens if babies are already being formula fed?

The decision to change the recommendations to suggest the introduction of solids at around six months came from a systematic review of research, which essentially showed that there was *no harm in waiting* until six months, but that this delay *might reduce infections*. The review was based on the combination of findings of two randomised controlled trials and 17 observational studies. Overall the review found that there was no difference in weight, length or head circumference at 12 months between babies exclusively breastfed for four or six months before introducing solid foods. This meant that timing of solids did not appear to slow down growth – babies were clearly still getting enough energy and nutrients to grow. However, babies who were introduced to solids at six months had fewer gastrointestinal infections, while their mothers lost more pregnancy weight (good in countries that have high levels of obesity) and also experienced a greater delay in their periods returning (great for most new mothers, but especially good for those in developing countries where childbirth is riskier and access to contraception poor).

There are several explanations for these findings. Firstly, increased infections may happen because solid foods are introduced. Introducing foods increases the risk of contamination from utensils, the preparation process, or the food itself. Solid foods also tend to displace breastfeeding, which means a reduction in intake of the protective antibodies in breastmilk. Overall, the expert panel convened by the World Health Organization agreed that *'the potential benefit to waiting until six months outweighs any risks'*, and thus the recommendations were changed.[6]

Some argued that the impact of reduction in infections was not long-lasting. Babies aged four to six months who had been introduced to solid foods might have had more infections than those who were being exclusively breastfed, but once that breastfed group received solids there was often no significant difference anymore.[7] However, even if this is the case, it is still important. If you can reduce the likelihood of small babies getting infections, even for a short period, and there is no other detriment – then that's still a great outcome!

However, research in the area continued. Some researchers (often, but not all, receiving funding from industry) were aghast at the change, believing that babies should still have solids from four months old. Long story short? They did lots of research. Other researchers who believed in the six months guidance did lots of research. Some who really had no preference did some too. What did they find? Most found that there was no real harm in waiting until six months. One almost comical review paper examined 33 different papers on the health impacts of waiting until six months and decided that 13 supported the idea, 13 suggested earlier and seven were neutral. Notably this work was funded by Nestlé.[8]

To be more specific, some studies have shown a protective effect of waiting until six months on respiratory infections. Others found evidence that waiting might reduce ear infections, digestive disorders and the risk of overweight. Lots, however, found nothing. But looking at the overall pattern, it was *rare* to find that an earlier introduction of solids was beneficial. For example, a systematic review looking at the timing of solid foods and child obesity found no clear link at 12 months old. Some studies showed babies who had an early introduction were heavier, while others showed no difference. A *very* small proportion show early introduction is associated with lower weight.[9]

So the recommendations to introduce solids at six months seem sound. Some disgruntled researchers have made statements like *'introducing solid foods at six months is at best neutral'*… which is not quite true, but even if it was, is still a great outcome. Breast and formula milk is high in energy and nutrients, so if babies are fine on this until six months then great – it's the quickest, easiest and likely cheapest way of getting calories into your baby.

What about allergies?

The association between the timing of starting solids and allergies is often in the news and is a complex subject. Some researchers insist that delaying solids until six months helps reduce allergy risk, while others want allergenic foods introduced from three months. Some suggest that in recent years (since solids have been delayed) the allergy rate has increased and this is causal evidence that the two must be linked.

However, lots of other things have been linked to the increase in allergies, including vitamin D deficiency, lower intake of fruit and vegetables and higher fat intake. The genetic case is also strong for allergy: if one identical twin has an allergy there is a 67% chance the other will as well. Genetics can't explain the rapid changes in allergy levels, but it could be that our environment is triggering genetic risk that was always lying there in wait. Finally, there is the hygiene hypothesis, which I am very drawn to (as it lets you cut down on cleaning) – that we are over-sanitising our environment and as a consequence children are not getting exposures that build the immune system.[10]

Finding firm answers about allergy has always been difficult, and in the past I've been known to say to students that 'no one quite knows', which although it may sum up the situation, isn't terribly satisfying. To try to get to the bottom of it for this book I looked at more than 100 research papers on timing of solids and allergies. And I'm *still* at 'no one quite knows.' Depending on which side you want to argue for, you can find numerous studies that show protection from delayed introduction, protection from early introduction, or nothing much. Unfortunately, what this means is that the research can be cherry-picked for unsuspecting audiences.

Delving into the literature, many studies looking at the impact of timing of solids on allergies show no impact. And lots of those that do show an impact at 12 or 24 months actually find, when they follow children up later on, that the differences have disappeared.[11] Another thing to remember is that although studies might be 'statistically significant', the real-life difference to the individual might be impossible to quantify. Someone dealing with the health costs of an entire population is in a very different position to someone looking at the individual risk to a particular child.

One problem in allergy research is that different studies look at different things – some look at introducing *any* food, while others look at the most allergenic foods. Some look at introducing to children with a *family history* of allergy, others look at *all* children. Some consider only *food allergies*, while others look at *any allergies*. The wording can be misleading: some studies talk about 'early introduction', but actually mean the introduction of allergenic foods at around nine months! These studies have looked at 'earlier introduction' compared to when many parents introduce allergenic foods. This is totally different from looking at the timing of introduction of any solids.

Much of the work on allergy is correlational – researchers look at when parents chose to introduce foods and then look at allergy risk. But there are many other things that can predispose a child to allergy. An awful lot of abstracts of papers on allergy risk include the sentence 'the strongest predictor of allergy was family history'. Further, if you have a family history of allergy you may well decide to leave off introducing solids as long as you can, especially if you are breastfeeding. However, genetics often 'win', and your child ends up developing an allergy anyway. This can mean that the research appears to show that delaying solids can 'cause' allergies.

The proof of the pudding (pun intended) is often in the detail of the research. Studies might explore specific allergies that have very low rates in the general population. One study, for example, claimed that introducing wheat after six months increased the risk of wheat allergy. But in the entire sample of 1,600, only 16 developed a wheat allergy, with only four children actually having positive blood tests.[12] Another study suggested early introduction of fish based on 16 out of 2,614 children having an allergy.[13] In both these studies, family history rather than just timing was a major predictor of whether an allergy developed.

A *lot* of allergy research is funded by industry, which means that you need to tread carefully. Beware the abstracts and read the findings. One Nestlé-sponsored paper I found had an abstract that reads *'there is mounting evidence that delayed introduction of commonly allergic foods is at best neutral and may be detrimental'*,[14] completely ignoring the studies *cited in the paper* that showed a protective effect! We've also already seen that 'at best neutral' is actually a good outcome.

Two recent randomised trials are often cited by proponents of early weaning as showing the need for early introduction of solid foods. The LEAP study randomised babies aged between 4 and 11 months who were at high risk of allergy (because they already had eczema or egg allergy) to avoid or consume peanuts. Those in the consume group were given small tastes of peanut spread over three or more meals a week (about 6g in total) until they reached five years old. The avoid group were told not to introduce peanuts until five years old. Those who ate the allergen did have a lower risk of developing allergy than those who did not (1.9% versus 13.7%), which suggested a protective effect for peanut consumption on peanut allergy in high-risk children.[15]

The EAT study also randomised babies to have small amounts of allergenic foods from three months of age alongside continued breastfeeding, but looked at all babies rather than just those at high risk of developing allergy. Another group breastfed exclusively for six months. The researchers found that when comparing the two randomised groups there was no difference in allergy levels. However, when they compared only those who actually gave the recommended amount of allergenic foods to their baby (rather than those who were randomised to do so) to those who exclusively breastfed, there was a small protective effect of early introduction on risk of peanut and egg allergy, although the overall percentages experiencing these allergies were low. The peanut group represented a 2.5% occurrence versus 0%, and the egg group 5.5% versus 1.4%.[16]

However, there are some issues with the EAT findings. Only 42% of babies in the early introduction group actually received the full amount of allergenic foods, with the researchers noting it was challenging to encourage babies this young to consume enough of the target foods. Levels of breastfeeding were also very high, suggesting the results may only apply to breastfed babies. In the early introduction group, 97% were breastfeeding at six months, and in the standard group 98% did so. This is far higher than the general population figure in the UK of around 34% at six months. It is plausible that mothers who signed up to this study are different in other health-related behaviours compared to the general population.

Another issue is that although these trials show a potential protective impact of early introduction, other studies do not. For example, one randomised controlled trial that looked at delaying the introduction of cows' milk until one year (compared to normal behaviour – many parents introduce cows' milk at around six months in cooking or in the form of yogurts and cheese) found that later introduction was associated with a reduced risk of cows' milk allergy at two years of age.[17] Another intervention study that asked mothers to avoid common allergens during pregnancy and breastfeeding, and then delay introducing them, found that this reduced the number of allergies at 12 months compared to those who carried on as normal.[18]

Interestingly, breastfeeding may be a mediating influence on the development of allergy, and a number of researchers who lean towards early introduction of solids nevertheless emphasise the importance of not stopping breastfeeding (the EAT and LEAP study authors, for example). Several studies found no impact of timing of solids on allergy risk, but did find that exclusive breastfeeding offers protection over partial or no breastfeeding.[19] Others have highlighted the effect of breastfeeding during the introduction of solids on subsequent allergy risk.[20]

For example a review of a number of research studies showed that babies who are breastfed through the introduction of solids have more than a 50% reduction in the risk of developing coeliac disease. It is thought that breastmilk helps the baby tolerate the introduction of an allergen better. There are a number of possible explanations for this. If breastmilk intake is high, the amount of solids consumed is lower, meaning that there is less exposure to the allergen. Fewer gastrointestinal infections – which breastfeeding protects against – may protect the digestive system. Further, the antibodies in breastmilk may mature the gut lining or reduce inflammation caused by the introduction of the allergen, soothing the whole process.[21]

Some studies suggest that there may be a window for gluten introduction at around six months. Early introduction was associated with a large increase in risk, while later introduction (after seven months) was associated with a slight increase in risk compared to six months. However, not all studies have confirmed this 'window', and the risk of early introduction was far higher than the risk of late introduction.[22]

The findings from these studies are certainly interesting, but have not as yet changed the guidance on introducing solid foods. Exercise caution, and if you are wondering about your family's particular circumstances, you should discuss them with a health professional.

Is milk really enough until six months?

Breast or formula milk is high in energy and has the right balance of energy and nutrients that babies need until around six months. Introducing puréed solids before six months displaces milk and contains fewer calories and nutrients, actually reducing the quality of a baby's diet. Breastfed babies will get fewer valuable antibodies and other factors found in breastmilk. Milk should continue to be an important part of the diet and WHO recommends breastfeeding to two years and beyond. Any solid foods introduced should logically be given for a reason: to increase nutrient intake (particularly important for iron and vitamins), to provide a good source of energy, or to introduce new tastes and textures. Of course the overall plan is to wean your baby from breast or formula milk eventually, so they do need to get used to eating foods, but the process is a marathon, not a sprint.

Babies who are formula fed should consume around 600ml a day of formula milk during the period when they are introduced to solid foods at 7–9 months, decreasing to around 400ml at 9–12 months (although the formula manufacturers may suggest higher volumes). For breastfed babies it is not such an exact science. But babies under a year old continue to get a big chunk of their nutrition from breast or formula milk. Breast and formula milk have around 67–69 calories per 100ml, providing at least three-quarters of a baby's fat and protein requirements, and at least half of the carbohydrates, in the second six months of life. Cows' milk is not a suitable replacement for breastmilk or formula milk at this stage, as it has a high protein content, a higher amount of some minerals and is low in iron. After one year whole animal milk can become the main milk drink if babies are not being breastfed.

A common worry is that breast milk becomes insufficient in some way as a baby gets older. This isn't true. Generally speaking, breastmilk will contain enough nutrients to exclusively breastfeed a baby until six months. This includes iron and zinc. As we have seen, babies are born with stores of certain minerals, such as iron and zinc, and gradually use these up over the first few months, being 'topped up' by minerals in breastmilk or added to formula. By about six months these stores are running low, so the baby needs to start eating solid foods, which contain nutrients such as iron in greater amounts.

Another concern is the difference in content between breast and formula milk. Breastmilk is lower in a number of nutrients than formula milk. This does not mean breast milk is deficient. Nutrients in breastmilk are absorbed differently. Formula milk is regulated by law and has to contain nutrients in sufficient quantities – due to the different levels of absorption this means including them in larger amounts. For example, babies will absorb 80% of the zinc in breastmilk, but only 30% of the zinc in formula milk (15% from soya formula). Iron is similar: babies will absorb around 50% of the iron from breastmilk, but only 20% of that found in formula. Thus the levels of these minerals in formula have to be higher so that babies get the right amount.[23]

One study found that babies exclusively breastfed for six months had a lower iron intake than those breastfed for four months with solids then introduced alongside breastfeeding. The four-month group had higher iron levels than the six-month group. However, there was no significant difference in the groups when it came to those who were low in haemoglobin – actually anaemic – suggesting that total iron intake alone does not determine iron status.[24]

The human body is very efficient and will try to protect breastfeeding mothers from deficiency. If we look at iron, breastfeeding contracts the uterus after birth, reducing the risk of haemorrhage. Continued unrestricted breastfeeding delays the return of periods (reducing iron loss) and breastfeeding women absorb more iron from food than women who aren't breastfeeding. Breastfeeding also appears to mobilise iron from the mother's iron stores more easily than when she is not breastfeeding.

One exception is evidence that a large proportion of the population in the Western hemisphere is deficient in vitamin D, especially by around April when we have come through winter. The risk is exacerbated among pregnant and nursing mothers. This is partly because we are aware of the damaging effect of too much sun and tend to stay out of it, cover up, or use sunscreen, meaning we do not get enough vitamin D. Generally speaking we need around 30 minutes of sunlight on our skin each day to produce sufficient vitamin D. I don't know what the weather is like where you are reading this book, but where I live in Wales…? No chance. Mothers who are deficient in vitamin D are less likely to produce breastmilk with sufficient vitamin D. However, a randomised controlled trial showed that when the mother was supplemented with vitamin D, her baby received sufficient supply.[25] Since 2003 it has been recommended that all breastfeeding women in the UK take a 10μg/day vitamin D supplement.

More than just timing

The WHO guidelines about when and how babies should be introduced to solid foods are extensive.[26] It is about more than when. Complementary foods should be:

1. Timely

Foods should be introduced when they are needed – when they offer something over and above what milk feeding can offer. We will look at this in more detail later, but breast or formula milk offers sufficient nutrients and energy for the first six months of life. Thereafter, a baby's stores of minerals start to drop and the levels in milk are not sufficient to replace them. Therefore they need solid foods containing these nutrients. As solid foods will displace milk in the diet, they should not be given unnecessarily early. Milk is a high-energy food, and breastmilk contains antibodies and other crucial bioactive substances. The need for additional nutrients must outweigh the benefits of a milk diet.

2. Adequate

Babies have energy and nutrient needs that must be met from the diet. Many of these can be gained from milk, but not all. Therefore additional foods should meet these needs. If a baby needs iron, they need iron-rich foods – not to be filled up with carrots.

3. Safe

In the West we are lucky to be able to prepare safe foods in clean conditions. However, we still need to take care to avoid infections by preparing foods properly (e.g. cooking through if necessary, freezing and thawing appropriately, not leaving jars of baby food open too long). Feeding utensils should be properly cleaned.

4. Properly fed

This means giving solid foods in response to a baby's signals that they are hungry or full. Babies should be offered sufficient food, but not too much. We should be aware of babies' age, skill level and general health. Where babies can self-feed they should be given the opportunity to do so.

Responsive feeding

In addition, the WHO stresses the importance of responsive feeding. Babies should be offered enough food, but not too much. They should be allowed to be active in their feeding, and have their feeding and satiety cues met. Babies should not be left hungry, nor encouraged to overeat. The WHO lists specific attributes of responsive feeding:

- Feed with a balance between giving assistance and encouraging self-feeding, as appropriate to the child's level of development

- Feed with positive verbal encouragement, without verbal or physical coercion
- Feed with age-appropriate and culturally appropriate eating utensils
- Feed in response to early hunger cues
- Feed in a protected and comfortable environment
- Fed by an individual with whom the child has a positive emotional relationship and who is aware of and sensitive to the individual child's characteristics, including changes in physical and emotional state

In other words, introducing solids to a baby is about more than what you give them – how you give it is important too. The feeding experience is also about more than just nutrition: relationships and the wider environment are important too. We will look at this more closely later in the book.

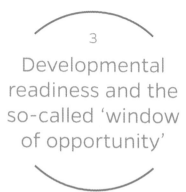

3

Developmental readiness and the so-called 'window of opportunity'

The guidance on introducing solid foods at around six months is primarily based on health evidence, but also takes into account a baby's physical development. Introducing solids at six months is a significantly different experience from introducing them at four months, because babies are developmentally ready not only to receive food, but also to participate in the process.

'Developmental readiness' means looking at how babies' physical development – both internally and externally – can inform us about when they should receive complementary foods. On a simple level, this theory suggests that when a baby is ready to feed themselves solid foods… they are ready to feed themselves solid foods! However, to be able to self-feed a baby needs to mature through a series of stages. Just as babies learn to hold their head up, roll, crawl and walk – predominantly as a consequence of developing control over their own muscles – they learn to eat solid foods. And just as in other stages of development, as long as babies are given the opportunity to develop as expected, most will get there in their own time. For example, the majority of babies learn to walk eventually, and this is predominantly determined by their own internal abilities rather than us 'teaching' them. There is no need to think that eating solid foods would be any different.

Babies are seen as developmentally ready for solid foods when they meet a number of key milestones. These milestones are all generally met between four and six months of age. In some babies they may start to occur a little earlier, but most babies will have met them by around six months. Some occur sooner than others (the tongue-thrust reflex disappears at around four months, for example, while another indicator – being able to sit up without support – doesn't generally occur until around six months).[1]

These milestones don't just apply if you are thinking about going down a baby-led weaning route (more on that later), but for giving all solids. There is a big difference between being able to swallow some food presented by an adult and being truly physiologically ready to self-feed. It is possible (although certainly not advisable) to give babies that are just a few weeks old solid foods, if you persist long enough with small enough amounts. However, just because you can, doesn't mean that you should. Think about it – when you eat you like to sit upright and put food in your own mouth at your own pace. Babies are no different. They do not like being fed in a reclined position, or having food repeatedly spooned back into their mouth if they push it out.

The first indicator of developmental readiness is being able to *sit up well with support*, which the majority of babies do by around six months. This allows the baby to remain in an upright position the whole time they are eating – and to concentrate on the food rather than trying to stay upright! Some consider babies ready for solid foods if they can sit with support, perhaps in a highchair – the key factor is really whether they can sit well for long enough without being reclined. Look at their posture – would you eat in that position?

The second indicator is that the *tongue-thrust reflex has disappeared*. Babies are born with a reflex to push anything (apart from a nipple) out of their mouth with their tongue, presumably to protect them from putting things – or having things put – in their mouths while they are still young. The reflex disappears between four and six months in most babies. It is easy to spot. If you put purée into a baby's mouth and they push it back out, that is the tongue-thrust reflex in action. It is often seen as 'cute' or 'funny', and there are countless videos on YouTube of babies doing it. It is neither cute, nor funny – it is a sign that the baby is too young to have solid foods. The body has developed a protective mechanism, which disappears once a baby is ready to eat solid foods. Why would you override that? Why would a baby need solid foods, while still having a reflex that made it difficult for them to eat?

Next on the list is the *ability to pick things up and put them in the mouth*. This is quite a complex series of events, and it takes a good few weeks for babies to be able to coordinate properly. I remember watching my oldest when he was about eight weeks old. He suddenly became aware of his hands, which seemed to be attached to his arms, which were attached to him. He stared at his hand for a good few minutes, then moved it ever so slowly through the air (still staring intently), before making contact with the toys in front of him. The look of shock on his face was fantastic and he continued to repeat this experiment, becoming more and more excited.

Similarly, a baby has to coordinate many movements to get something from tray to mouth. At first they will use a palmar grasp – sweeping something up into the palm of their hand to pick it up. This usually comes at around four to six months. By nine months they are likely to have progressed to a pincer grip and be able to pick up small things. It is likely that these stages are protective and match a baby's developing ability to control foods in the mouth. A palmar grasp allows bigger objects (foods) to be picked up to chew and suck on, while a pincer grip allows foods like peas to be picked up. These are foods that if not managed correctly in the mouth might slip to the back and be swallowed whole.

This leads us to *mouth control*, which also develops in stages. Babies are born with the ability to suckle on the breast. This is quite a specific set of jaw and tongue movements. They can also suck and swallow from a bottle. Sucking is fine for liquids, as chewing is not needed. However, with solid foods babies can no longer just suck them in and swallow at the same time. They need to learn to use the tongue, jaw and teeth if they have them (teeth are not needed for solid foods; the gums and jaw work perfectly well).

Once the baby has all these skills they are ready to self-feed. Most babies acquire these skills between four and six months of age. Meanwhile, internally, babies' digestive systems are developing to be able to digest solid foods properly. This also varies between babies, but generally happens at around four to six months. See where I'm going with this? Babies develop externally to self-feed at about the same time they develop internally to cope with that food. It's as if Mother Nature intended it...

Of course, we cannot see how a baby is developing internally. Researchers looking at developmental readiness have noted that external signs may be present in some babies before six months old and this might suggest that they are ready internally too. However, you cannot see inside a baby to check this and given that the evidence suggests that there is no harm in waiting until six months to introduce solid foods, it seems logical to wait until six months to be sure that your baby is ready internally as well as externally.

If you want to read about this in more scientific depth there is a great (but complex) review paper by Naylor and Morrow entitled 'Developmental Readiness of Normal Full Term Infants to Progress from Exclusive Breastfeeding to the Introduction of Complementary Foods'.[2] The paper itself is as long as its title suggests, but notes several key points to support the concept of babies being ready for solids once they can self-feed, including:

'the majority of normal full-term infants are not developmentally ready for the transition from suckling to sucking or for managing semi-solids and solid foods in addition to liquids until between six and eight months of age'

and

'Using the available information on the development of an infant's immunologic, gastrointestinal and oral motor function, as well as maternal reproductive physiology... the probable age of readiness for most full-term infants to discontinue exclusive breastfeeding and begin complementary foods appears to be near six months or perhaps a little beyond...'

and

'...there is probable convergence of such readiness across the several relevant developmental processes.'

In other words, the baby goes through a series of developmental stages, both in terms of internal digestive ability and external physical feeding skills. In most babies, by around six months these combine to enable babies to self-feed and digest food. Magic!

Is there a 'window of opportunity' for solids?

One concern parents often have when they hear that babies should not be introduced to solid foods until six months is 'missing the window of opportunity'. They may have heard this phrase from someone who believes that babies should have solid foods earlier. The 'window of opportunity' view reflects the opinion that babies *must* be introduced to solid foods by around six months or 'bad things' will happen (such as feeding difficulties, fussiness and weight loss). It sees introducing solid foods as a learning/teaching process rather than a natural, developmental process, which it is the responsibility of the caregiver to encourage.

However, the evidence for 'bad things' happening is pretty limited. Firstly, why would something that is essential for survival (eating) be something that we need to learn? We don't get taught or learn to breathe – we just do it. Physical skills such as walking are acquired as we slowly develop control over our muscles. Most babies don't need 'teaching' to eat and will simply do it in their own time, no matter how much we might like to think we are enabling them to be 'advanced'.

Secondly, until around 1940 (and the rise of the baby food industry) babies didn't get introduced to solid foods until around 11–12 months. Further back in history children didn't really eat solids until after they were weaned at around three years old. Yet there is no record of serious feeding issues in the population. The concept of progressing through stages: breastmilk, milk food, purée, lumpy foods, family foods…

was essentially created by the baby food industry in order to sell a wider range of products.

There is some evidence that shows an *association* between a delay in solid foods and feeding issues, but there is no research that shows *causality*. One paper that is widely referred to is Illingworth and Lister, 1964.[3] They showed a link between babies not *'learning to chew'* at six months and later feeding issues and concluded that *'if a baby is not given solid foods shortly after he has learned to chew, there may well be considerable difficulty in getting him to take solid foods later'*. The abstract for their paper states:

> *'Children should be given solids to chew at a time when they are developmentally ready: in an average child this age is 6 to 7 months. If they are not given solids then (as distinct from thickened feedings, which can be given any time after birth), they are very apt to be difficult about taking them later, failing to chew, refusing the solids, or vomiting.'*

However, a little digging into the research shows that the majority of the children observed had learning difficulties or physical disabilities, which probably led to both a delay in introducing solids and feeding difficulties – rather than the delay causing the difficulties. Just because two things happen together does not mean that one necessarily causes the other.

A more recent study showed a similar pattern, finding that babies who were not given lumpy foods until after 10 months were less likely to be eating family foods at 15 months. However, this was not a randomised controlled trial of the timing of introduction of solids, but an observational study. It is likely – given that the data were collected prior to 2001, when the guidance was to introduce solids at four to six months and the majority of babies had solids by four (if not three) months – that if a baby wasn't eating lumpy foods by 10 months there was a wider issue around feeding or development happening.[4]

Meanwhile, other evidence fails to show a link between later introduction of solids and fussy eating, and my own research on timing shows that later introduction (albeit not after six months) is associated with less fussy eating and better appetite control in toddlers.[5]

Dr Gill Rapley, author of several baby-led weaning books and a researcher in the field, also makes a very valid point about the observation that if you introduce solid foods to older babies they are more difficult to spoon-feed. She states:

'What is rarely acknowledged is that spoon feeding provides a means whereby semi-solid food can be inserted into the mouth of an infant too immature to achieve this for himself. Seen in this light, the response of the older infant can be interpreted as the reasonable actions of an individual who is sufficiently physically mature to make his wishes plain, whilst the 'acceptance' of the younger infant becomes simply evidence of his inability to resist'.[6]

But my baby won't eat!

Just as with other stages of physical development, all babies are different. Some are raring to go at six months; others are less interested. In my personal 'sample' of three children I had one developmentally ready by around five months, one who tucked in heartily at six months and another who was far more gradual in getting round to actually eating something. I remember my anxiety about whether he was ever going to eat food. Would I have to breastfeed forever? Of course he eventually ate and does so perfectly well now.

Try to ignore the scare stories and remember that introducing solid foods is about gradually moving from a milk diet to a solid diet. *Slowly.* Tastes and textures are more important than amounts. Keep offering. Some babies accept solids more readily than others and this may be genetic. We know that there is a series of genes involved in babies being more particular about foods.

Introducing new tastes takes time, especially if they are not sweet. Babies often need to be offered a food several times before they decide to trust it enough to eat it – this is a protective instinct. It stops them eating anything and everything they come across in the wild. Numerous experiments with fruit and vegetable purées have shown that young babies may need 8–10 exposures to a new taste before they accept and enjoy it. Bitter-tasting vegetables might take even longer. Interestingly, one study showed that eating a wide variety of tastes might help – babies who had a more varied diet accepted novel foods more readily.[7] So if your baby doesn't seem to want a food, don't force the issue. But try again a few days later. Persistence will eventually pay off!

If you are worried about your baby's weight or how much they are eating, speak to your health visitor or GP. Remember that as long as they are still having lots of breast or formula milk, they are still getting nutritious food.

Overall, look at your baby's development and ability to manage foods. Offer suitable foods to help them master the different skills needed for eating. Provide the right environment and they will naturally do the rest. At their own pace.

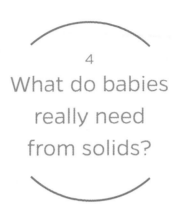

4
What do babies really need from solids?

One of the biggest concerns new parents have when introducing solids is the concept of getting 'enough' into their baby. Enough energy, enough nutrients, enough tastes… the list is endless, and of course there are the vague yet dire warnings you may hear about babies 'needing to get onto solids ASAP at six months' or 'breastfed babies not getting enough iron or zinc'.

I spent a lot of time exploring what babies *actually need* for this chapter. It didn't make sense to me that, given what we know about babies' natural stages of development and therefore readiness to start eating solids during the second part of the first year, and the historical trends showing introduction of solids at closer to a year, that babies would suddenly become hugely deficient and doomed to terrible things if they didn't start eating lots of solids at six months precisely. Nature simply wouldn't design babies this way.

This isn't a 'how to' book that will tell you to give your baby proteins, carbohydrates and fats at set times, or a recipe book (for those, see the further reading section). But I do want to explore babies' specific needs a little. When the guidelines say that you need to give them protein, how much protein is that? How much energy? And what nutrients? I was pleasantly surprised to discover how small those specific needs are... and how relatively easily most babies get them. Now this is not to say that introducing a wide range of foods isn't important – but the concept of the first few months of solids being about exploring new tastes, textures and smells is very valid. This isn't about filling your baby up with as much solid food as possible. Breastmilk does not lose all its nutrition at midnight on the 180th day. Formula milk has energy and nutrients in it. Your baby will still be getting these. Adding solids is about *complementing* these – which is why starting solids is often called giving *complementary* foods.

Yes, your baby needs to start moving from a milk-based diet to one where in the future they will be eating family foods. But there is no need to panic and rush your way through the process. It's important to understand what the real point of introducing solids is, and the best foods to meet those needs. I willingly admit that I didn't understand some basic principles back when I was introducing solids to my children – and I don't think we do enough to teach new parents about this now. There is guidance about which first foods are suitable, which foods to avoid and suggestions about how to feed. But do we understand the rationale behind the guidance? Or how much (little?) our babies need?

As breast or formula milk remains a major source of energy and other macronutrients (protein, fats, carbohydrates) for your baby until 12 months old (breastfeeding can of course continue beyond 12 months for as long as you and your baby like, but there's no need to fork out for formula after 12 months because your baby can have regular full-fat cows' milk), the last thing you want to do when introducing solid foods is reduce their milk too much. When babies are first introduced to solids they tend to replace milk intake with food. They do not take in more energy overall. This is a critical point given that many people want to introduce solid foods because they perceive their baby needs 'more'. A bit of carrot purée is not going to miraculously fill your baby up and make them sleep through the night.

Thus, thinking about the foods you want to give your baby is important. Very simply, the foods you offer should be *more nutritious* than breast or formula milk. They should provide *additional* nutrients or energy. Fruits and vegetables are important in terms of vitamins and minerals, but are also low in calories and high in bulk – displacing higher calorie milk. This explains why some babies become more 'unsettled' at the start of weaning, wanting more milk feeds. Of course, fruits and vegetables are also important, because they will add new tastes and textures to the diet, but the focus should be on more nutrient-dense foods at first.

So how much energy do babies need from solid foods? Until nine months babies need less than 200 calories a day from solid foods – the bulk should still come from milk. That's not even four Jaffa cakes. (Don't feed your baby Jaffa cakes! Eat them yourself.) The point is that 200 calories isn't much. It certainly doesn't reflect the amount of pressure that parents feel to ensure their babies are getting 'enough'.

The next sections look at what babies really need, with an emphasis on reducing worry. Try not to focus on what your baby gets every day – think of their diet as a pattern over a week or so.

How much energy do babies really need from solid foods?
Babies are small compared to full-grown adults, but in terms

of energy requirements they need far more per kilo of body weight than we do. The average female adult, for example, needs around 2,000 calories a day, and according to the Office of National Statistics, 'Ms Average' now weighs 70 kilos. A baby born weighing less than 5% of her weight needs around 25% of her calorie intake. From birth to three months, a baby needs around 124 calories per kilo of body weight per day. If we as adults ate that, Ms Average would need nearly 9,000 calories a day. That's a lot of cake!

Babies need more energy because they're growing – by the time they reach six months old, they'll have doubled their birth weight and then tripled it by one year. They don't continue growing at this rate, or they would be (even more) challenging to cope with as teenagers. Boys need a little more energy than girls, mainly because they tend to be a little heavier and grow a little faster. The following table from the World Health Organization guidelines on introducing solids shows approximate calorie intakes for babies during the first year – as they age their calorie intake needs per kilo of body weight drop.[1] These figures are approximate, and different sources give slightly different numbers (e.g. in the UK First Steps Nutrition Trust publishes its own figures). But all sources suggest similar amounts.

Energy needed during the first year in kcal/day

	Boys	Girls	Per kg body weight
0–3 months	545	515	124
4–6 months	690	645	116
7–9 months	825	765	109
10–12 months	920	865	103

As we have seen, the change from a milk diet to a diet of solid foods should be gradual. The following table from the

World Health Organization shows how that change should roughly occur. As you can see, the amount of calories needed per day from solid foods is really quite low until babies are around nine months old.

Remember that this is a guide and that the amounts are estimates across those age ranges. For example, you wouldn't suddenly start giving your baby 200 calories on the first day of solids and then on the day they reach nine months nearly triple it. It's about slowly moving from milk to solids, reducing (or displacing) milk bit by bit.[1]

From	solid foods kcal/day
0–3 months	0
4 –6 months	0
6–8 months	196
9–12 months	455
1–3 years	779

These calories from solid foods should be split across mealtimes, aiming to move towards three 'meals' a day by around eight months. The portion sizes will look very small – and for more guidance on portions First Steps Nutrition Trust has some great downloads, split by age of baby. It can be really helpful for parents to 'see' how much food is a baby-sized portion.

Purées, finger foods or a mix?

Traditionally (by which I mean how you were probably introduced to solid foods), babies were introduced to puréed foods first, followed by a range of textures until they were eating normal family foods. 'Finger foods' were included along the way. The World Health Organization recommends that babies start with purées and that finger foods are introduced from eight months.[2] The UK Department of Health says that babies can have both purées and finger foods from the start of weaning.[3]

The vast majority of parents choose to introduce first foods in purée form. Findings from the last UK Infant Feeding Survey (2010) found that 96% gave foods that had been puréed or mashed to start with. Fifty-seven per cent of babies had baby rice as a first taste, with a further 10% given rusks.[4] The NHS in the UK suggests:

> *'Your baby's first foods can include mashed or soft cooked fruit and vegetables like parsnip, potato, yam, sweet potato, carrot, apple or pear, all cooled before eating. Soft fruits like peach or melon, or baby rice or baby cereal mixed with your baby's usual milk, are good as well. Finger food is food that is cut up into pieces big enough for your baby to hold in their fist with a bit sticking out. Pieces about the size of your own finger work well. Your baby learns to chew this way. Try grabbable bits of soft, ripe banana or avocado.'*

These are great suggestions, but there are no set rules – although you should avoid foods that are a choking risk such as nuts and whole grapes, and honey due to the small risk of infant botulism. There are lots of baby recipe and weaning books that can give good ideas – but there is no evidence to suggest which are the 'best' foods for longer-term health. What you should focus on are sources of good nutrition, rather than calories that will simply fill your baby up.

What about nutrients?
Aside from energy intake, there are guidelines for the different types of nutrients needed. It is important to remember that

these nutrients will come from both milk and solid foods, and that breast or formula milk can provide a good chunk of many of them. Again the emphasis should be on making a gradual move to a solid diet.

You'll also likely be pleased to know that research looking at babies' intake (based on diet diaries) shows that, generally, babies get enough nutrients. One study in Canada looked at intake up to 12 months and found that, apart from vitamin D and iron (more on these later), most babies were meeting their intake needs. They also tended to increase the amount and variety of foods they were eating from the start of solids until 12 months – so remember, if you have a six-month-old taking very little, that everything will probably have changed by their first birthday.[5]

There are two types of nutrients: macronutrients, which are fats and proteins and carbohydrates, and micronutrients, which are vitamins and minerals and fibre. It is important to consider both when introducing solid foods. In general, milk is good for providing macronutrients, but less good at providing micronutrients. This does not mean that milk is somehow 'lacking': micronutrients should come from solid foods.[1]

Fats

Fats often get a bad name, especially with media scare stories about childhood obesity. However, fats are needed for healthy growth and development. They are an essential part of the diet, offering energy, essential fatty acids and the fat-soluble vitamins A, D, E, and K. Babies should get 35–45% of their total energy intake from fat. However, not all fats are the same. There is plenty of fat in a fast-food meal, but no one is suggesting babies should develop a drive-through habit! Dietary fats can be split into visible fats, such as cooking oils, and 'hidden' fats in products, and are made up of fatty acids. Most of the fatty acids in animal fat – such as cows' milk and meat – are saturated. Plants and fish are more likely to contain monounsaturated or polyunsaturated fats. Unsaturated fatty acids are considered a better choice for everyone over the age of five, but breastmilk has a high saturated fatty acid content as well as some important unsaturated fatty acids, all of which are needed for development.

One of the best sources of fat for babies is breastmilk, with around 50% of the energy coming from fat. The fat in breastmilk is made up of 98% triglycerides, which are the richest source of energy at 9 calories per gram. There are also two essential fatty acids that the body cannot make itself: linoleic and linolenic acid. These are used to make other fatty acids including arachidonic and docosahexaenoic acids. Babies find it difficult to make (and pronounce) these fatty acids – so breastmilk contains them and some are added to formula.

Protein

Protein has a positive reputation, and as adults we often hear about diets where 'high protein' is linked to ideas about lean muscle and weight loss. Babies definitely need protein, but too much can be a bad thing. High intakes of protein in infancy can lead to too much growth and overweight.[6] In the right amounts, it is a vital part of a baby's diet.

Proteins are essential for the function and structure of all the body's cells. They make up parts of the body – such as fingernails and hair – and are involved in the production of hormones. Protein is particularly important in the early years due to rapid growth. The body only holds small reserves of protein (about 3% of body content) and therefore a regular supply is important. However, young babies actually need less protein per kg of body weight than adults. An intake of 5–6% of the overall diet is recommended for babies, compared to 10–15% for adults. The recommended protein intake per day is about 13.7g per kg of body weight at 7–9 months and 14.9g per kg of body weight at 10–12 months.

This is a fairly easy nutrient to give to a baby though. If breast or formula milk intake is significant, from a protein perspective little else is needed. Milk is a very good source of protein – the most protein-rich foods are breastmilk and eggs.

Carbohydrates

Carbohydrates are one of the main sources of energy. They are converted to glucose, which is used by all body tissues and particularly the brain, which can't metabolise fat for energy. Providing energy is a key focus of complementary feeding. Sources of carbohydrates include sugars (which babies love, but which provide no other nutrients) and starches. Sugars can be divided into naturally occurring sugar (e.g. in milk as lactose, and in fruit and vegetables) and added free sugars (e.g. sugars added at the table, in recipes, or in soft drinks). The sugars in fruit juices, smoothies and fruit purées are considered to be free sugars. The general population is encouraged to have a diet which has no more than 5% of energy from free sugars, and in some areas it is recommended that free sugars are not given in the first year of life.

Starches provide energy and are found in foods such as potato, other starchy roots, cereals, breads, pasta and rice. They are usually well tolerated, but they are quite bulky, meaning that babies eat smaller quantities and take in fewer calories. High-fibre carbohydrate foods should not be given to babies because they are bulky and slow the rate of digestion, meaning babies don't take in enough calories. Some high-fibre foods also contain phytates, which impair the absorption of iron and zinc. However, fibre is important for good digestion and babies will get plenty if they have a good intake of fruits and vegetables.

Micronutrients: vitamins and minerals

Babies need a range of different vitamins to help them grow and develop. Different foods offer different nutrients. For example berries and citrus fruits are a good source of vitamin C, while wholegrain cereals offer a range of B vitamins. Offer your baby a wide range of foods and do not worry too much about the individual micronutrients. Breast and formula milk will still offer some of these nutrients too. For example, a typical intake of breast or formula milk will give your baby almost all the vitamin A they need, and lots of vitamin C, alongside the more obvious things such as calcium.

Remember to look at patterns of eating over a week, rather than a day. As we've seen, most babies are getting a wide enough range of nutrients. The baby food industry would have you believe that it is incredibly difficult to get these nutrients into your baby, but this isn't true. A healthy diet with variety is all that's needed. In some circumstances a vitamin supplement may be appropriate, and this can be discussed with your healthcare provider.

Vitamin D

Breastmilk and many foods are low in vitamin D, because humans make vitamin D from the action of sunlight on the skin. Thirty minutes of summer sunlight on your skin daily should give you enough vitamin D and the same goes for babies. However, many countries in the northern hemisphere do not get enough sunlight for this to happen, and parents are concerned about their babies getting sunburned and either avoid the sun or use sunscreens, which can reduce exposure. It is therefore recommended that breastfed babies have vitamin D drops from birth, and that formula-fed babies have them if they are taking less than 500ml formula (which has added vitamin D) per day. This is one vitamin recommendation that the evidence very much suggests should be supported.

Iron

Stories and advertising in the media have meant that many parents are now concerned about their babies' iron levels. Advocates of early weaning and formula companies cite babies' iron needs as something that parents need to worry about. Is this true?

Iron deficiency is one of the most common nutritional issues in young children and worldwide 43% of children under the age of four suffer from iron deficiency. The majority live in developing countries where complementary foods sources are limited in variety or nutrient-poor. All babies need to be offered iron-rich foods from six months, as their stores are depleting, leading to a drop in haemoglobin levels and eventually anaemia. Anaemia in children under the age of five years old is defined as a blood haemoglobin level of 11.0g/dl or less (10–11g/dl is mild, 8–10g/dl moderate and below 7g/dl severe).

With iron, the amount *consumed* and the amount *absorbed* are very different. On average, only around 10% of iron consumed is actually absorbed by the body, and this varies across foods. There are two types of iron in food: haem iron and non-haem iron. Haem iron is in meat and oil-rich fish and around 25% is absorbed by the body. This is not affected by the presence of other dietary components. However, most people get the majority of their iron from non-haem sources. This is particularly true of complementary foods, which often contain little meat. Consuming meat and fish actually helps iron from vegetables to be absorbed – when meat is added to a meal, the absorption of iron from vegetables increases by 50%.[7]

The amount of non-haem iron absorbed by the body also depends on the body's stores. If you are iron deficient you will absorb more of it than if you are not. It also depends on what you eat with it – vitamin C may help absorption, while foods such as unleavened bread, whole grains and cheese can reduce it. Tea reduces iron absorption by nearly two-thirds, which is one reason why it is not recommended as a drink for young children.

Iron is stored in the body to some extent. When you eat iron, some is used and some is stored. At birth babies usually have large iron stores, which are gradually used up over the first six months while they are exclusively breastfed. However, if the mother has severe iron deficiency (< 7g/dl) the baby's store could be low – although moderate deficiency (8–10 g/dl) doesn't seem to affect the baby's stores. Iron stores are also affected by the amount of blood transferred from the placenta to the baby at birth, before the umbilical cord is cut. Waiting to cut the cord therefore helps ensure that the baby has adequate iron stores. Preterm babies are at greater risk of iron deficiency because they are smaller, so their stores are smaller. They also use more in catch-up growth after they are born.[8]

Babies need iron for a number of reasons. Firstly, for rapid growth during the first year – and there is some suggestion that babies who grow very rapidly might have bigger iron needs.

Secondly, we all lose small amounts of iron through turnover of cells. Babies fed unmodified cows' milk before six months are at risk of losing iron through damage to the intestine – this is one of the biggest risk factors for iron deficiency.

For the first six months iron should come from breast or formula milk. After that it should come from the diet. Health authorities recommend that babies should be given iron-rich foods from the start of complementary feeding, such as eggs, meat, fish and pulses, rather than relying on the iron in milk. Note that the amount of iron the body needs is far lower than the amount that needs to be consumed, because only around 10% will be absorbed. Babies need to absorb about 0.55mg of iron a day – which they will get from an intake of around 7mg.

Formula is fortified with iron to a higher level than breastmilk (despite the recommendation that iron should come from complementary foods). Some (those that sell formula milk) claim that breastmilk is 'low' in iron, but this is biologically normal – iron is supposed to come from a varied diet, not from milk, just like vitamin D is supposed to come from the sun. Formula manufacturers would have us believe that breastmilk is deficient, but offering your baby a wide range of nutritious foods alongside continued breastfeeding is nutritionally optimal. Iron in breastmilk is very well absorbed at 50% (compared to 20% in formula), meaning that babies breastfed for the first six months will have sufficient iron based on intake (around 0.2mg absorbed per day) plus some from the iron stores they were born with.[9]

If you are still concerned, baby vitamin drops can be given, although most in the UK only contain about 2mg per day with about a 10% absorption rate – giving around a third of the requirements. Add in breastmilk (another third) and you still need some from food. There are low levels in vitamin drops for a reason – excess iron can do significant damage to babies. Iron is poorly absorbed by the body and bacteria thrive on iron. If lots is being consumed but not absorbed, it is the perfect food for any bacterial infection. Excess iron can also cause diarrhoea. Iron toxicity in babies and toddlers can cause damage to the heart, lungs and liver. Iron is an excellent example of why 'more' is not necessarily 'better'. This is one reason why most everyday foods are not fortified with iron – because of the risk to men and postmenopausal women of excess intake (which has been linked to heart disease).

Calcium

Breastmilk contains less calcium than formula milk. However, again absorption rates are important. Human milk averages 200–340mg calcium per litre, but 67% is absorbed. Infant formula, on the other hand, has roughly 510mg per litre, but less is absorbed, meaning actual absorption rates are comparable. Of course, formula manufacturers don't put that on the tin. Interestingly, giving mothers calcium supplements does not increase the amount in their breastmilk. This is because breastmilk is not deficient – the calcium in it is meant to be at that level.[10]

What about getting too much?

As we've seen, the majority of babies do get enough macro and micronutrients. Often without their parents measuring it too much. However, too much of any vitamin can be a bad thing. Excess amounts will often not be absorbed and simply excreted (particularly with vitamin C, for example), but significant overdoses can cause harm. Although you would have to be consuming quite a lot, over-consumption of vitamin A, for example, can lead to jaundice, nausea, loss of appetite, irritability, vomiting and even hair loss. It is very important never to give vitamin supplements that have not been recommended for your baby, or to give more than the recommended dose.

Research has also shown that although most babies are getting what they need from food, some are fed non-nutritious foods. One study showed that 5% of babies aged 4–5 months have sweetened foods such as desserts or sweetened drinks daily, rising to 17% at 6–8 months, 43% at 9–11 months and 72% at 12 months.[11] In one study, more than a third of the increase in energy intake between six months and four years came from sweets and soft drinks.[12] Remember that any food that displaces breast or formula milk should be nutritious. These foods are not good replacements. Occasionally, yes. Every day, no.

What about follow-on milks marketed from six months?

Formula milks fall into three categories: first stage or infant milks (suitable for 0–12 months), second stage or follow-on milks (6–12 months) and third stage (toddler milks). Follow-on milks are often promoted (by those who market them) as an important part of a baby's diet. But are they really needed?

Short answer – no.

Slightly longer answer – still no. Infant and follow-on formula milks have pretty much the same ingredients. There is absolutely no need to move your baby from infant formula to a follow-on formula. You can keep them on infant formula until 12 months and then they can move on to regular full-fat cows' milk. Nobody apart from the follow-on manufacturers thinks they are a good idea. The World Health Organization, the NHS and the American Academy of Pediatrics all recommend that babies stay on infant formula.

Follow-on milks are basically the same as infant milks, but with some vitamins and minerals included at higher levels. However, this is unnecessary – the whole point is that your baby is starting to eat complementary foods from which they can get these vitamins and minerals. Secondly, there isn't *that* much difference. Looking at a comparison in nutrient content between infant and follow-on milk, both have similar energy and protein levels. Infant milk has slightly less carbohydrate, but since the most popular first foods are often carbohydrate-based I wouldn't worry about this. Fat is actually a little higher. Levels of vitamin D and zinc are pretty much the same. The only real difference is in iron. Follow-on formula has twice as much. But again, babies should be getting iron from complementary foods as it is better absorbed. Also the difference in iron between infant and follow-on milk is approximately the amount of iron in vitamin drops. Vitamin drops cost about 10p a day and many parents are eligible to receive them free through the Healthy Start scheme.

Research into follow-on milk has not found any advantage to growth or development over infant formula.[13] In fact, there is even a suggestion that overly fortified follow-on formulas may harm development. Infants in Chile given these milks had lower cognitive and learning outcomes at age 10.[14]

What if I'm breastfeeding – does follow-on milk have more nutrients than breastmilk?

No. The manufacturers would like you to think it does (and they use slogans to induce anxiety). If you are breastfeeding you can carry on to meet the milk requirements of your baby's diet. Breastmilk provides energy, protein, fat and calcium – all the energy and nutrients your baby needs from a main milk drink. It was not designed to be packed full of different vitamins and minerals such as iron. Those come from the baby's stores, and from complementary foods when ready. The advice from all organisations is that the additional requirement for nutrients should come from complementary foods, not 'special' milks.

The ingredients in follow-on milks are not magic. They include modified cows' milk, vegetable oils (including palm oil), vitamins and minerals and some added bits you already get in breastmilk. Breastmilk may not have the added vitamins and minerals (because they are meant to come from the diet), but it does have many other important bioactive substances that your baby would not receive if you stopped breastfeeding. These include antibodies, which are abundant in breastmilk. The evidence suggests that these antibodies are particularly protective while you introduce your baby to solid foods, helping to guard against allergic reactions and contaminants.

The cost of swapping from breastmilk to follow-on milk is significant. Babies of 6–9 months are recommended to have three 200ml bottles a day. Giving your baby this formula from a tub would cost 90p per day (based on a 900g tub costing £9 lasting about 10 days), or you could pay 75p each for ready-made cartons, costing £2.25 daily. Comparatively, breastmilk is free and sufficient alongside solid foods. If you really want to give vitamin drops they cost about 10p per day. Comparing over a month that's either free (breastmilk), £3 (breastmilk plus vitamin drops) £30 (follow-on formula) or £70 if you're going for ready-made follow-on formula.

Why does follow-on formula even exist?

Follow-on formula was invented by manufacturers because infant formula cannot be advertised directly to families in many countries. In the US, where there are no advertising restrictions, there is no follow-on formula. Globally, follow-on formulas generate around £10 billion in profit every year. In 1981 the World Health Organization launched an International Code of Marketing of Breastmilk Substitutes, which encouraged countries to ban the promotion of breastmilk substitutes for babies under six months old.[15] The Code supports:

> 'the provision of safe and adequate nutrition for infants, by the protection and promotion of breastfeeding, and by ensuring the proper use of breastmilk substitutes, when these are necessary, on the basis of adequate information and through appropriate marketing and distribution … if babies are not breastfed, for whatever reason, the Code also advocates that they be fed safely on the best available nutritional alternative. Breastmilk substitutes should be available when needed but not be promoted'.

The 1981 Code and subsequent WHA resolutions up to 2016 say that formula milks for babies under six months should not be promoted. Manufacturers were told not to advertise the products, use money-off deals, use promotional stands, give free samples or contact pregnant women. All educational information should state the superiority of breastfeeding. This applied in all countries that adopted the Code. In 2016 a resolution clarified that a 'breastmilk substitute' included all products marketed in the first three years of life. However, this resolution has yet to be adopted by many Member States, including the UK. So in many countries follow-on formula can be marketed, and the branding means that it is often mistaken for infant formula advertising. The companies also promote a natural progression through their products, using stages and numbers on products to suggest you should move through them in turn.

You might think that if companies blur the lines between infant and follow-on milk, brazenly marketing to parents with a baby under six months, that this would be a Code violation and therefore illegal. You would be right. Currently it is difficult to do anything about it, however, as the companies are clever, have big budgets, and know that the regulations are often not enforced. Baby Milk Action collects examples of misleading or Code-violating marketing and works to hold the companies and the regulators accountable (for details, see Chapter 9).

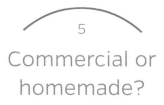

5

Commercial or homemade?

The evidence, emotions and politics behind food choices

A quick glance at the baby food aisle in any supermarket will tell you that commercial baby food is big business. Parents often have questions about whether the food they offer their baby should be commercial or homemade, and the vast majority of parents use commercial baby food at some point – and this has been true since the rapid expansion of the baby food industry in the 1930s. However, how much commercial baby food is used varies considerably, and there is comparatively little research exploring whether it really matters or not. This is interesting, given that public health authorities stress the need for an evidence base for self-feeding (baby-led weaning). When you dig a little deeper it becomes clear that the evidence base for much common practice (the need for puréed foods, the difference between commercial and homemade food) is equally scanty.

In reality, the choice about the type of food your baby gets is not as straightforward as it sounds. Family budgets, availability of foods, the wider family diet and cultural preferences all influence feeding decisions.

There is also the underlying question of whether babies even need special baby foods rather than eating the family diet. The sheer scale of the baby food business – and the politics and economics behind it – is vast, but is it necessary? Amy Bentley, in her book *Inventing Baby Food*, describes how, when she was first introducing solids to her baby, she realised that jars of apple purée for *babies* had exactly the same ingredients as regular jarred apple sauce, yet were hugely more expensive per gram. Compare further the cost of an apple to the price of a small jar of puréed apple – it is vastly more expensive. Our desire to give our babies 'the best' lines the pockets of the baby food manufacturers.

Are commercial baby foods sufficient?

Commercial baby foods need to stick to some compositional standards. In Europe this is covered under a directive by the European Commission for 'cereal based foods and baby foods for infants and young children'. This regulation is currently being reviewed and new compositional guidelines are expected after 2018. Baby foods are subject to general food laws, and there are standards for hygiene in preparation, use of food additives, presence of contaminants and the use of materials that come in contact with the food.[1] There are also guidelines for some minimum/maximum nutrient levels, although these vary slightly in the UK/EU and USA, while the World Health Organization has its own guidelines. The figures should therefore be seen as approximate, but baby foods should contain roughly 12% protein, no more than 31% fat and no more than 57% carbohydrate.[2]

One study in the UK looked at the macronutrient content of eight ready-to-feed baby meals. They found that all the products had at least the minimum protein levels. Those containing meat had on average 23% protein, while those containing vegetables had 16%. The average energy density was in line with breastmilk. However, although most foods were within the fat content range, two vegetarian meals exceeded the limit because of the inclusion of cream, cheese and whole milk powder. The authors noted that this was concerning, as parents often perceive vegetable-based products to be 'healthy' and 'lower fat' choices.[3] A study in the USA looked at the sodium content of 657 baby foods, finding that all but two were low in sodium.[4] Meanwhile, a study in Norway examined the concentration of minerals and trace elements in a range of different baby foods and found that all were within the upper limits. Toxic elements were very low – which is good to know![5]

It should also be noted that family meal choices are not always healthy. One study in the UK explored the sodium intake of eight-month-old babies, finding that 70% of the sample consumed excess sodium. Although this data was collected in 1991/2 and sodium limits for baby foods have now been reduced, the greatest contributors to excess sodium were bread and cows' milk (for those babies who had transferred to cows' milk as a main drink). Only 20% of sodium came from baby foods. Bread may have up to 200mg of sodium per slice – so two slices can take a baby over the upper limit. Cows' milk has almost double the sodium of formula milk and three times that of breastmilk. Gravy is another suspect – just one tablespoon can have 150mg. Also, beware 'baby' versions of adult foods. One study found that the average baby yoghurt contained more sodium than adult versions.[6] Another study analysed multiple products labelled as baby versions and found that cereal bars, fruit snacks and yoghurts all had more sugar in than the adult versions.[7]

Context also matters. In one study, infants of low-income mothers who received infant food packages containing baby food fruits and vegetables consumed a significantly greater variety of fruit and vegetables than those whose mothers did not.[8] If you are on a very tight budget and cannot afford a wide range of foods for your baby, commercial foods may be an affordable way of introducing more expensive food tastes such as mango or strawberries.

What are the drawbacks to commercial foods?

As with any food, it is usually not a good idea to only eat pre-prepared products. Commercial foods differ in taste and texture from homemade foods. Industrial machines make purée far smoother than any homemade version, and the processing increases the sugar content of the food. As babies start to learn about textures and tastes, variability is important. Home-prepared foods usually taste a bit different from meal to meal – and that is a good thing. If you are aiming to present your baby with a range of textures and tastes, commercial foods should just be part of a wider diet that includes home-prepared foods too.

Although research shows that commercial baby foods have sufficient levels of nutrients, some have too much of some ingredients, particularly sugar. Research from Glasgow University looked at all the different infant foods that were marketed in the UK. They identified 479 products, the majority (79%) of which were spoonable foods. Of those that were labelled as suitable from four months, 65% were sweet foods, although this proportion decreased as the suggested age range increased.

Looking at the overall nutrient content of all the baby foods in terms of energy, protein and carbohydrates, the average energy density was almost identical to breastmilk, with slightly lower sugar levels. However, when the sweet foods alone were considered, the sugar levels for spoonable foods were double that of breastmilk, and provided far less fat and energy. When dry finger foods and snacks were examined, these foods had over three times as much sugar as breastmilk. Those snacks that contained fruit contained *over five times as much sugar* as breastmilk – 31.8g of sugar per 100g. Snacks that contained no fruit still contained nearly four times as much sugar as breastmilk – and given the absence of fruit that must mean added sugar. If babies are eating a high proportion of dry foods – including rusks – their level of sugar consumption is likely to be far higher than is recommended.

Babies are predisposed to like sweet foods, so it is in the manufacturers' interests to provide them. Babies are likely to accept these foods, encouraging parents to continue buying them. In evolutionary terms sweet foods were a good source of energy, and our hunter-gatherer ancestors would have prized these rare treats highly. However, added sugar did not exist. Sugars came from fruits and vegetables – alongside vitamins, minerals and fibre. As biological evolution takes so long to catch up with social evolution (and our associated food stocks), babies are still programmed to favour sweet tastes. However, taste preferences can develop in the early months and be long-lasting, so it is an ideal time to introduce other important flavours.

The Glasgow study also compared the average nutrients of commercial foods versus a homemade equivalent. The average ready-made meat/fish/chicken baby food had half the level of protein of a homemade version, with the same pattern for vegetarian equivalents. Sugar-wise, rusks have 10 times the sugar content of a slice of toast with butter. Energy content is typically higher in home made 'main meal' food compared to shop bought (up to double the kJ), while sweet foods tend to be far higher in energy when commercial. A rusk, for example, has four times as much energy per 100g as a banana. Thinking about where the energy comes from, those that are high in sugar are most likely to have their energy from this, while those that are lower in sugar (e.g. main meals) are more likely to have it from fats.[9]

These are not isolated findings. A study in the USA found that around half of foods that were grain-fruit mixes had added sugar and over 35% of calories from sugar, while two-thirds of dairy-based desserts contained added sugar and over 35% of calories from sugar. Notably, healthy sounding 'vegetable purées' contained on average 40% of their calories from sugar. Although you would expect fruit purées to be high in sugar, one-fifth had further added sugar.[10] Thus, babies who consume more commercial foods have higher overall intakes of sugar.[11] Another study in Europe calculated the nutrients that would be consumed if only commercial baby foods were used, finding that the amount of protein in the diet might be too high, especially if babies were also formula fed.[12]

Portion size is a significant issue. A report by First Steps Nutrition Trust found that the portion sizes recommended for many commercial baby foods exceeded the recommended amount of energy that babies should be eating from solid foods. The report found that 61% of products for babies aged 7–9 months and 86% (savoury) and 90% (dessert) for those aged 10–12 months exceeded estimated energy requirements. At the same time, many of these commercial foods were lower in energy density than is recommended: they had fewer calories for the bulk of food being consumed.[13] Babies need to eat a larger amount of less energy-dense foods to get enough calories, but this is often difficult or even impossible given their small stomachs. Trying to encourage a baby to eat more than they need may cause them discomfort and break down their ability to regulate their appetite properly, increasing their risk of overweight (more on this later).[14]

Further, the content of commercial baby food does not always match the description on the packaging. One study looked at baby foods that had fruit and vegetables in their names. Although some contained high quantities (up to 94% – notably none were pure fruit), some contained as little as 13%. In fruit products, often very little of the ingredient named on the packaging was included, for example, apricot (11%), strawberry (10%) and raspberry/blueberry (5%). Foods labelled apple and pear contained much more of the named fruit, (45% apple, 37.5% pear). For vegetables the top contents were for mixed veg (34.5%), tomato (28.5%) and cauliflower (28.5%), while the lowest were swede (12%), broccoli (8%) and red pepper (7%).[15]

On that note, beware vague marketing phrases like 'a source of'. How much do they mean? Likely very little. Also, just because something says 'no added...' doesn't mean there is none in there. It means there is none added... so a food can still be high in sugar and salt, as long as it is naturally occurring. And natural doesn't necessarily mean good. Under EU law baby foods must contain 10% or more of an ingredient to be able to include that ingredient in the name of the product. Just 10%.[16] That means that a 'chicken and vegetable dinner' can be just 10% chicken and 10% vegetable. Call it a 'vegetable and chicken dinner' and it need only contain 8% chicken! This means that jars and pouches often contain a high proportion of vegetables and water, making the product less nutrient-dense and meaning that larger quantities must be consumed to obtain the levels of nutrients.

Finally, high levels of commercial food consumption might alter dietary preferences in the long term. One study found that the more commercial foods a baby ate, the higher their diet was in added sugar in preschool and primary school. This doesn't necessarily mean that there is a direct link – although given the high levels of sugar in commercial foods and learning experiences of babies there is a plausible connection.[15] Another study found that the higher the intake of commercial food a baby had, the lower their consumption of fruit and vegetables in preschool and primary school.[17]

Is home cooking safe and sufficient?

Parents may worry that if they make their own baby food they might prepare it incorrectly or somehow accidentally poison their baby. Marketing has a lot to do with this – when baby foods were first introduced they were advertised based on the fear that nutrients were destroyed and bacteria introduced in home cooking.

One novel study explored whether foods made by a manufacturer were any less contaminated than those made at home. A baby food manufacturer supplied samples of a product alongside its recipe. The food was recreated in lab conditions and mothers were asked to prepare a version at home. No differences were found in the final products for energy, fat, carbohydrate, protein, or a series of vitamins and minerals, apart from zinc being higher in the homemade version. Although the commercial version had the lowest bacterial growth, all samples were microbiologically safe. Notably, at least one sample of peaches in all groups tested positive for pesticide residues – although these were well below residue limits.[18]

Do I need to follow a fixed plan?

There are a number of baby food writers who try to persuade parents that introducing solids is a military exercise, involving exact amounts and combinations of food at set times. They tend to recommend freezing food in ice-cube trays and thawing and heating specific numbers and combinations of cubes for meals, and require lots of baby-food-making paraphernalia.

Books can contain interesting ideas for food combinations, and can help you think about preparing foods for your baby if you want to take a spoon-feeding/puréeing approach. They will probably have information about preparing and cooking foods and safely freezing them. But do you need to give set amounts at set times of set foods (some of which you have likely never heard of?). Probably not. There is no research to suggest that babies need this sort of structure. But if you find this sort of approach reassuring, carry on – there's also no evidence of any harm.

What about organic?

Many parents worry about whether the food they give their babies should be organic. Fears about pesticides in food and their impact on babies is common, and organic food makes up around 10% of all baby food sales. Are these concerns justified? A study in 2012 that analysed hundreds of foods found no evidence in favour of organic foods.[19] Other things like vitamins and minerals, and offering a range of tastes and textures, are arguably far more important than whether the food is organic or not. And although organic food must have lower levels of traceable pesticides, the limit for allowable traceable pesticides in baby foods is so low anyway that this really makes little difference. One study compared organic and non-organic baby foods and couldn't find any pesticides in either.[19]

However, many parents continue to worry and the baby food companies play on this anxiety. There is certainly no harm in buying organic – as long as you buy a range of different flavours… but be aware that many organic options are significantly more expensive.

The tricks of the baby food industry

Although manufacturers try to convince consumers that they really care about the health and development of babies, their main aim is to sell their products. They know that these products are more expensive than normal family foods, so they pour huge sums into promotion to appeal to parents and outperform their competitors.

If a country is following the WHO Code in full, baby foods cannot be advertised, unless they are for babies of six months or older. Follow-on milks, bottled water, juices, teas, cereals and any other baby foods should not be promoted as suitable for babies under six months as breast or formula milk is sufficient and the most nutritious option until then. Packaging should also be different to avoid cross promotion of brands.[20] Guidance suggests that:

> *Foods for infants and young children should not be promoted unless they meet all relevant national, regional and global standards for composition, safety, quality and nutrient levels. All processed food products for infants and children should meet applicable Codex standards and guidelines. National nutrition standards should be developed to define which products are appropriate for this age group, with a particular focus on limiting the added sugars, saturated or trans-fat, and salt content. Products within the scope of the Code should not be promoted'.*

Any food promoted for infants should support optimal feeding and avoid inappropriate messages. Specifically, messages and labels should include:

- A statement on the importance of exclusive breastfeeding for the first six months and of continued breastfeeding up to two years or beyond
- A recommended age of introduction (this must not be less than six months) and a statement on the importance of not introducing complementary feeding until about six months of age
- An appropriate ration/serving size consistent with complementary feeding guiding principles
- Nothing to suggest use for infants less than six months (including pictures, milestones, wording, images, illustrations, numbers, stages and bottles or teats)
- No information or image to undermine or discourages breastfeeding or suggest that the product is equivalent or superior to breastmilk
- Nothing that undermines or discourage appropriate complementary feeding or includes any pictures or text which may suggest that commercial products are superior to home prepared foods

Of course, industry tries to get around all this in inventive ways (as it does with formula milk advertising), exploiting to the letter the legislation and regulation in different countries. In the past, before the Code, manufacturers went much further in their advertising. Gerber baby foods, for example, were renowned for their emotional advertising slogans:

'It isn't fair to baby to spend long hours in the kitchen – for baby's sake and for your own learn what doctors tell young mothers just like you'

'You can't with ordinary home equipment prepare vegetables as safe, as rich in natural food values, and as reliably uniform as ready-to-serve Gerber products'

'If you've had to exchange a charming wife for a tired mother who spends endless hours in the kitchen dutifully scraping, stewing and straining vegetables for your child – you'll be glad to read this story.'

When research in the 1970s started to question the need for specific commercial baby foods, and more and more parents were choosing homemade, one manufacturer in the US, Beech Nut, wrote a letter to new parents to try to scare them into continuing to buy their products. They made reference to a very rare form of anaemia that was caused by ingesting huge amounts of nitrates found naturally in spinach and carrots, suggesting that babies were at risk if foods were homemade. The letter stated:

'Dear mother, we at Beech Nut feel obligated to advise you that some potential dangers for your child exist in home preparation of baby food…. Beech Nut as a responsible corporate citizen feels compelled to speak out in an interest of safety and nutrition for your baby'.

The letter backfired and a group of mothers sued the company. Although the case was settled out of court, Beech Nut had to send a second letter to all parents stating that home cooking was safe.[21]

These days manufacturers are more subtle in the ways they try to promote their products, though they constantly try to push the boundaries of the legislation. An example is in the labelling of foods as suitable from four months: in

Europe the manufacturers get away with this because not all of the provisions of the WHO Code, which is advisory to all countries, have not fully been put into law in the UK or other member states. Despite the fact that the Code was always meant to apply to companies as well as countries, the practice continues. Lobbying by health organisations, charitites and NGOs has so far failed to change UK legislation, although baby food company Organix has just announced that in future no foods will be labelled as suitable from four months:

> 'We're changing the labels on our stage 1 fruit pots and cereals to show they're suitable from 6 months+ in line with WHO and health department guidelines about when to start introducing solid food to your baby. These foods were previously labelled as suitable from 4 months+ and while babies can safely eat some foods at this age, we want to support families in line with national guidance so that we're not giving mixed messages. Breastmilk will provide enough energy and nutrients for growing and developing babies until they reach six months of age. Babies are rarely developmentally ready for solid food before about six months of age and the same advice applies to babies who are mixed fed or solely formula fed.'

This is important. Researchers explored what mothers in Australia and New Zealand thought about labels on baby food jars that said '4–6 months'. Most said that they felt this meant that they should introduce them at four months.[22] Health professionals are often asked by parents why the guidance is to introduce solid foods at six months but the jars on the shelf say four months. They feel that evidence-based health messages are being undermined by industry, and you can see why.[23]

What manufacturers display on their packaging can also influence choice. One study found that putting a wholegrain symbol on the front led parents to choose it as a perceived healthier option, despite it potentially having high levels of sugar.[24] This is common on savoury biscuit snacks for babies.

Advertising of commercial solid foods doesn't just affect what foods babies get – it can affect timing of introduction and duration of breastfeeding too. One study traced the impact of infant food advertising starting in St Vincent in the Caribbean in the 1970s. Until that point very little advertising was seen on the island and the majority of mothers used a combination of breast and bottle feeding. However, after the advertising campaign it was found that the more mothers could recall the adverts, the earlier they stopped breastfeeding.[25]

As we've already seen in relation to follow-on milk, people recognise products across brands, even when they've only been shown one, meaning that manufacturers can market a product for older babies, but people perceive it as an infant product, or make the link in their own minds thanks to brand recognition. Dr Nina Berry, a researcher in Australia, has shown in many studies that parents think they have seen infant formula being advertised, despite the fact that they live in a country that does not allow infant formula adverts. They perceive a product aimed at an older child as one suitable for a younger one. In one study mothers, grandmothers and health professionals were asked to identify formula milk products. Only 1 out of 19 correctly identified a toddler milk as a toddler milk.[26] In previous work, only 3 out of 15 mothers correctly identified toddler milks, with most mistaking them for infant milk. Mothers said that they usually just noticed the brand rather than reading the specific information on packets.[27]

Formula and baby food companies are of course very aware of this effect. In 2007 regulatory changes in the UK required formula companies to make it clear to parents that there was a difference between their follow-on milks and infant formulas. One study tracked what happened in terms of advertising. The results showed that despite a statement about suitability for babies over six months appearing alongside age recommendations on the packets, suggesting that the companies were following the rules, marketing campaigns were in fact stepped up. Adverts became more common and more widely distributed. Moreover, there was a greater emphasis on brands, more inclusion of emotions and more claims about health benefits. Meanwhile the products were still commonly seen as infant milks – over two-thirds of respondents in one survey said they had seen infant milk being advertised.[28]

Similarly, a UK survey asked 2,000 women, pregnant or with a baby up to one year old, whether they had seen adverts for infant formula. Over half responded that they had and while most were aware that follow-on milk existed and was different, pregnant women were the least likely to know this. These women are the new target market for formula advertising.[29]

This type of advertising can affect the timing of introduction of solid foods, due to increased brand awareness and recognition. In the US, hospital discharge packs with free samples of infant formula are common. One Randomised Controlled Trial showed the knock-on effect these packs can have on later choices, by randomising women to receive the usual advertising pack versus a pack about infant feeding. Those who received the advertising pack did not breastfeed as long and introduced solid foods earlier than those in the other group.[30]

Do I need 'devices'?

In recent years the number of products on the market to help you feed your baby has hugely increased. What do you really need? If you are making your own purées, some kind of blender and plastic storage containers are useful. Bowls, spoons and bibs are good purchases. And possibly a highchair.

But a quick look online reveals that you can spend almost £1,000 on highchairs that promise to do all manner of things. One site has over 1,100 products listed under 'weaning', including 325 different options for weaning spoons. There are also a number of devices that claim to purée and bag food for the freezer (or squeeze it directly into pouches). There are mesh feeder nets that babies supposedly want to chew on, bowls that stick to the highchair tray, food warmers... Think carefully about these things. How can you clean them easily and safely? Are they really essential or are they designed to relieve you of your cash? Would you eat from a mesh feeder?!

Summary

Whether and how much you use commercial foods will depend on your personal circumstances. We know that most parents use commercial foods at some point, but given their very high sugar levels and the lower levels of other nutrients compared to many home-cooked meals, it's probably best to use them in moderation. Be aware that what is being advertised may not be the full story. Read the labels carefully rather than looking at the brand names, and prioritise offering your baby a wide range of tastes and textures. Maybe try some of the foods yourself – that way you'll know what you're giving your baby and whether those tastes and textures are what you'd choose for them to get used to.

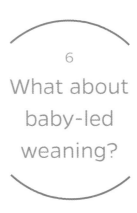

6

What about baby-led weaning?

As described in previous chapters, the second half of the 20th century saw an increase in popularity of infants being fed special 'baby foods', which were typically puréed and different to the family meal. However, more recently an alternative approach known as 'baby-led weaning' has grown in popularity. Instead of blending special foods and spoon-feeding them to babies, this approach encourages parents to offer their baby family foods, in their whole form, and allow the baby to self-feed. This means that babies can be part of family mealtimes right from the start of solid foods.

Gill Rapley, along with Tracey Murkett, published the first book on baby-led weaning in 2008.[1] Gill was a health visitor by background, who had seen the approach used by families and decided to investigate it for her MSc studies. However, discussion of baby-led weaning had begun before the book was published. I recently used social media to research where the term had first emerged, particularly in online communities, and found that discussion of the approach had started in around 2004, with an online forum developing, followed by Facebook groups. Google now returns around one million results for 'baby-led weaning' and some of the biggest social media baby-led weaning groups have over 150,000 followers. Why is it so popular?

As we've seen, guidance from the World Health Organization changed in 2003 to recommend that babies be introduced to solid foods at around six months of age rather than four. This meant that *how* babies were introduced to solid foods could also change. At four months most babies cannot independently sit up even with support, and some may not have strong head control. They are also only just starting to be able to coordinate picking up and mouthing objects. Their tongue reflex is also still present, meaning that they involuntarily push things out of their mouth to protect themselves from choking. Solids for a four-month-old must be puréed and given on a spoon.

By six months most babies can sit independently with support for a few minutes. They can pick things up and put them in their mouth. They can chew and swallow and their tongue reflex no longer pushes things out of their mouth. All in all, they are far better suited to being able to self-feed and do not require puréed foods in the same way. So the change in the recommendation about the timing of introduction to solid foods meant that the baby-led approach became a feasible way to introduce solids.

One study, actually entitled 'Is baby-led weaning feasible?' looked at a large cohort of babies in northern England and the age at which they were reported to have reached out for solid foods. They found that only two-thirds had done so by 4–6 months, but that 85% of babies had done so by 6–7 months and 96% had done so by 7–8 months. These figures were also thought to be an underestimation, as for a baby to be able to reach out to pick up a solid food, they had to be offered the opportunity by a parent. If parents were particularly anxious about the baby eating solid foods, did not want them to have finger foods or simply didn't offer them, then the baby would have been unable to do so and the answer on the survey would have been a 'no'.[2]

What does baby-led weaning involve?

There is no official definition of baby-led weaning. What we have are Gill Rapley's suggestions in the baby-led weaning handbook and a shared 'understanding' of the approach among groups on social media. With no body of evidence (as yet) suggesting that certain elements of baby-led weaning are particularly important, it remains open to individual interpretation. I discuss some of the central ideas below.

1. Allowing your baby to self-feed

In general, baby-led weaning involves offering the baby foods in their whole rather than puréed forms and allowing the baby to self-feed. One of the biggest 'discussions' (or in many cases full-blown social media wars), is about whether, if you're following baby-led weaning, you can ever purée a food or spoon-feed. Saying 'I'm doing a mix of baby-led weaning and purées' can lead to others denying that this is actually following a baby-led approach.

Does this matter? Research is starting to explore the question. From a research perspective, we simply don't know whether there is a 'magic number' of meals that should be self-fed to have any impact upon anything. However, we don't have any research evidence to support puréeing or spoon-feeding either. In terms of the baby-led weaning book and the members of online communities, most agree that a baby-led approach tends not to use spoons or puréed foods.

In my own research comparing a baby-led approach to a traditional puréeing approach, I have often asked parents how much they use spoon-feeding and puréed foods, and considered anyone using these 10% of the time or less to be baby-led weaning. This allows for real life… spoon-feeding when round at Granny's house with her new cream carpet, or for a yoghurt bought when out and about. However, recently we've come to realise that there seem to be three natural groups of those who say they follow a baby-led approach – those who never use spoons or purées, those who very occasionally use them and those who believe they are following baby-led weaning but use them quite frequently. So now we're exploring what the outcomes of these different approaches might be. Watch this space. And in the meantime, do what suits you and your lifestyle best.

2. Joining in family mealtimes and eating family foods

Other behaviours associated with baby-led weaning often seem up for debate. One of those is whether the baby eats family foods and joins in family mealtimes. Most research in the area suggests that babies who follow the baby-led approach are more likely to do this, but don't always at every meal. One study showed that in fact only around half of meal times were shared with the family.[3] This can be due to practicalities: for example, one parent getting home from work later than a baby might eat their main meal. Sometimes family foods are not suitable for babies, particularly if highly salted or processed.

3. Feeding responsively

A central underlying ethos of the baby-led approach is responsive feeding. As described earlier, responsive feeding involves letting your baby stay in control of how much they eat. No coaxing, pretending to be an aeroplane or making them finish meals. Baby-led weaning is responsive by its very nature. If a baby is self-feeding, then unless you are very persuasive in your language and they are very advanced in their understanding, you're not going to be able to get them to eat more! When we compared how responsive mothers were during the period they introduced solid foods to their baby, mothers who followed a baby-led approach were more responsive.[4] There is more on this in the next chapter, which considers why responsive feeding is so important however you introduce solids. I believe that the responsive feeding element of baby-led weaning is likely to be the biggest influence on any improved outcomes that research may show.

4. Delaying solids until around six months

Most studies show that babies who follow a baby-led approach are introduced to solid foods later than those who follow a traditional approach. This seems logical: for a baby to follow baby-led weaning they need to be closer to around six months old to be able to self-feed. It is highly unlikely that you would be able to baby-led wean a four-month-old baby. You could start offering them solid foods, but they would not be able to coordinate sitting up, picking up the food and getting it into their mouth.

It is possible that choosing baby-led weaning encourages parents to wait longer before introducing solids to their baby. However, it may also be that parents who are more likely to wait until around six months are more likely to be drawn to baby-led weaning. The BLISS study in New Zealand (BLISS stands for Baby-Led Introduction to Solids Study) randomised parents to follow either a 'usual' approach (in this case the majority chose a traditional spoon-feeding approach) or to follow a baby-led approach. Only 18% of those in the usual care group delayed solids until six months, compared to 66% in the baby-led group. As parents were randomised, this suggests that simply aiming to follow a baby-led approach delays introduction of solid foods to closer to six months.[5] This may have a positive impact on babies' later eating behaviour and weight, as a later introduction to solid foods is associated with lower risk of fussiness and overweight (as well as reduced risk of infections).

5. Milk feeding

Some suggest that baby-led weaning is more suited to babies who are breastfed. This is based on the rationale that babies who are breastfed have been more in control of how much milk they drink and when, and that breastfeeding responsively helps maintain milk supply. Mothers who have breastfed might find that a baby-led approach fits with what they've been used to, compared to those who might have fed to a routine or given set amounts at each feed. Most research studies in this area suggest that mothers who follow a baby-led approach are more likely to breastfeed, but this isn't the case for all.

If you are bottle-feeding and baby-led weaning, it is important to bottle-feed as responsively as possible (giving smaller amounts more frequently and stopping as soon as your baby shows signs of being full), as some studies show that bottle-fed babies are more likely to continue drinking the same amount of milk while they're being introduced to solid foods, whereas breastfed babies more naturally cut back. One reason for this might be the habit of preparing certain sized bottles and encouraging the baby to finish them, so be aware of this possibility.

What foods can be offered?

Generally, baby-led weaning works on the concept that

babies are capable of eating family foods from the start of weaning, and need little additional preparation of these foods. Developmentally, if a baby can pick up the food and place it in their mouth they should be able to manage to chew and swallow it safely. What is important is that babies are allowed to pick up the food and place it in their mouth themselves, as this will ensure that they naturally put it towards the front of their mouth, where they can then chew and manipulate it in order to swallow it. If you put food in a baby's mouth for them, it may go towards the back of their mouth, where they may swallow it before chewing it.

Having to pick up the food and place it in their mouth means that, to start with, babies will only be able to pick up larger food items. You can help by offering foods that have a 'handle', such as broccoli stalks, or that are a little bigger than the size of their palm so that they can scoop them up and still have some sticking out of the top. However, don't be put off offering your baby-led weaned baby spaghetti and sauce. They will devour around half and rub the other half all over their face, hair, highchair, the dog, the carpet, the walls…

Fascinatingly (or, you know, due to years of evolution) babies don't develop the ability to pick up very small foods like peas, that could accidentally be swallowed without chewing, until they are around nine months old. At this stage they develop their 'pincer grip', which is the ability to pick up a small item between their thumb and forefinger and put it in their mouth. They have also mastered the tongue and chewing skills to cope with these small items.

Lots of foods that you might not think are suitable can be given to a baby to self-feed. They don't need teeth – their gums are hard and do a pretty good job of demolishing food. Some foods won't be chewed and swallowed in their entirety; chunks of meat, for example, might be gummed and sucked.

For a detailed discussion of suitable foods see the baby-led weaning book or join one of the online groups.

Is there a choking risk?

The majority of foods should not pose a choking risk, as long as babies are allowed to feed themselves. Research that asked parents and health practitioners about choking risk found that mothers who follow a baby-led weaning approach rarely have concerns about choking.[6] Health practitioners have far more concerns.[7] Remember that there is an important difference between choking and gagging. Gagging is a normal part of learning to eat, whereas choking is a problem.

Choking occurs when the airways are blocked. A choking baby will often not be able to make much sound. They will likely be very distressed, grab at their throat or may turn blue. Choking will usually require a caregiver to intervene to force the food out of the airway. Gagging, however, is a normal reflex reaction for a baby learning to eat. Gagging happens when food moves to the back of the mouth and the baby coughs and splutters to bring the food back to the front of the mouth. Gagging is usually noisy, unlike choking.

Quantifying the frequency of choking is difficult. Parents must identify the difference between choking and gagging and then self-report how often it has happened. You can't follow babies around for months to see if they choke. The studies that have examined this asked parents whether their baby has choked or not. All studies have found no difference in choking rates by weaning group. However, choking is reported as common. In the BLISS trial, 35% of babies had choked at least once. Notably, a very high number had been offered a food that posed a choking risk: at seven months, 52% had been offered such a food and at 12 months, 95%.[5]

Research suggests that it is best to avoid hard apple slices, as small parts can snap and break off and be swallowed. The same goes for raw carrot sticks. Some research has shown that babies often get given foods that are generally unsuitable for small children, so avoid things like nuts and popcorn, due to the choking risk, but also marshmallows, as they can be swallowed and expand in the throat. Sausage slices can also be a problem, as they can be swallowed whole and stick in the windpipe. Whole grapes and cherry tomatoes should be halved lengthways (look online for how to do this). In several rare cases children have died from swallowing these foods whole, as they fit neatly into a child's windpipe and are smooth and difficult to extract.

Are all family foods suitable?

Generally, if you are baby-led weaning you will want to think about what foods you are offering your baby. Just because it is home-cooked or can be self-fed doesn't mean a baby should be eating it. Parents are often worried about spicy foods, but these are usually fine. Things to watch are salt levels, additives and saturated fats that might be acceptable for adults, but too much for a baby.

Parents often report that they modify their family foods to suit the baby better. However, one study asked parents to keep food diaries before and after introducing their baby to solid foods. Although this was only a small-scale pilot study, the researchers found that there was no change to the family diet in terms of macro or micronutrients before or after weaning. Moreover, analysis of the adult diet diaries found that their diets were higher in sodium and saturated fat content than both UK and USA guidelines. This is concerning, but the study also found that babies only participated in about half of all adult mealtimes, so this may not be such a problem.[3]

Does baby-led weaning encourage a better diet or
healthier weight?

Those who follow the baby-led approach often say that
they feel that the method helps babies to develop a range of
positive eating habits and helps them stay a healthy weight.
This is one of those areas where although we may feel there
are a number of plausible reasons why this might be the
case, the research has not yet caught up to give us definitive
evidence. Unfortunately, research into baby-led weaning
only started in the last few years and there have only been a
handful of exploratory studies conducted. One trial of a baby-
led approach is currently underway, but this is not enough to
be able to scientifically endorse the method.

Does it affect the diet eaten during introduction
to solid foods?

At present, only one study (the BLISS trial) has actually
compared the diets of babies following a baby-led or
traditional approach. Researchers used a three-day weighted
food record, which means they asked parents to weigh
everything they offered their baby, and what was left of it
afterwards, and record what and how much the baby had
eaten over the three days. They compared two groups of
seven-month old babies: 76 who followed the BLISS approach
and 71 who followed standard weaning. Babies in the BLISS
group were more likely to consume 'meat', 'cows' milk or dairy
products' and 'sweet foods', but were, surprisingly, also more
likely to consume 'powdered infant cereal'. Meanwhile, the
babies in the standard group were significantly more likely
to eat 'ready-to-eat commercial infant foods'. No differences
were found between the groups for consumption of 'fruit and
fruit juice', 'vegetables' and 'bread, pasta, rice and low sugar
cereals'.

The researchers then looked at the different nutrients consumed. There were no differences between the groups. Both groups got 10% of energy intake from protein, 45% from fat and 45% from carbohydrates. However, when the data was analysed excluding milk feeds, infants in the BLISS group consumed significantly more protein and fat. This may be because the inclusion of protein-rich food at every meal was encouraged as part of the intervention. For mineral intake, those in the BLISS group consumed double the amount of sodium and selenium and less vitamin A. The higher-than-usual consumption of sodium is a possible concern, but more research is needed.

Iron consumption is often an area of concern for parents introducing solid foods, especially in baby-led weaning, as babies might not be offered iron-fortified cereals or other foods. One of the key points of the BLISS trial was to encourage parents to offer their babies foods that were rich in iron, and a list of these foods and how to prepare them was given. This appeared to have a positive effect. In a pilot of the trial, mothers who were planning to follow a baby-led approach were assigned to simply follow their own version of baby-led weaning, or to follow the BLISS approach with its emphasis on iron-rich foods. Compared to the 'own version' baby-led group, the BLISS group babies got more iron-containing foods in the first week of introduction of solid foods, and were offered more portions of such food at six months (2.4 versus 0.8 portions a day).[8]

In terms of energy intake, again only the BLISS trial has measured this through food diaries. They compared energy intake at seven months and 12 months, but found no difference between the groups at either age.[8]

Does baby-led weaning affect later eating behaviour?

Research that interviewed both parents and health practitioners shows that both groups feel that the baby-led weaning approach may have a positive impact on future eating behaviour. Mothers who have followed the approach believe that it reduces fussiness and promotes better appetite control. Practitioners also believe it may expose babies to a wider range of tastes and textures, and help them learn to stop eating when full. However, the studies, particularly those with mothers, rely on the perceptions of those who have successfully followed the approach, rather than measuring any outcome in children's eating behaviour.

Two studies have explored whether later eating behaviour is affected by method of introducing solid foods. One study asked mothers at 6–12 months how they were introducing solid foods to their child, and then at 18–24 months asked them to rate their toddler's eating behaviour. It specifically asked about fussy eating and how well children were able to control their appetite (e.g. stop eating when full). It found that toddlers who had followed a baby-led approach were less likely to be rated as fussy eaters and more likely to be rated as able to control their appetite compared to those who had followed a traditional approach. However, this was based on mothers reporting their child's eating behaviour rather than a measure of their intake.[9]

Another study looked at pre-school children's food preferences (as reported by their mother). This found that children who had followed a baby-led approach had a greater preference for carbohydrates, whereas those in the traditional group had a greater preference for sweet foods. However, this study simply asked parents to recall whether their child had followed a baby-led weaning approach or not. Differences were very small.[10]

Does baby-led weaning affect weight?

Again, only a few studies have compared the weight of children who followed a baby-led or traditional approach. In the longitudinal study described above, there was no difference in weight between the baby-led and traditional group at birth or at six months. However, those who had followed a traditional approach were heavier than the baby-led group at 18–24 months, by just over 1kg on average. Looking at weight group (e.g. underweight, normal weight, overweight), 86.5% of those who followed a baby-led approach were normal weight, 8.1% overweight and 5.4% underweight. In comparison, 78.3% of those who had followed a traditional approach were normal weight, 19.2% overweight and 2.5% underweight. The difference in numbers in the overweight group was significantly different. However, this was a very small percentage overall and, importantly, all weights were self-reported by the mothers.[9]

The study that examined pre-school children also collected data on weight. Again, the average weight of children who had been traditionally weaned was greater than those who had followed baby-led weaning. However, over 80% of children were a healthy weight, and some weights were self-reported.[10]

Finally, the BLISS trial weighed and measured babies at 6, 7, 8, 9, and 12 months to compare differences between the two weaning groups. At the time of writing the full data has not been published. However, initial findings reported show that no child experienced growth faltering, but 32 babies experienced slow growth (but not by clinical definitions). However, there was no significant difference in slow growth between the two groups.[11]

Can we be sure any impact is to do with self-feeding family foods?

Certainly many parents and supporters of the baby-led approach feel this is true and there are a number of reasons why this might be the case. For example, we know that delaying solids, continued breastfeeding, responsive feeding and home-cooked foods can all help to build healthy eating habits and weight, so it is feasible that lots of different elements of the baby-led approach might be positive. However, more research is needed to test this. Some of the reasons why baby-led weaning might be a positive thing outside of the self-feeding of finger foods aspect are:

1. Because they were introduced to solid foods later

As noted previously, babies who follow a baby-led approach start solids significantly later on average compared to those following a traditional approach. Starting solids later is often associated with a lower risk of overweight. Therefore this in itself might be a protective element of the approach.

2. Because they were more in control of how much they ate

A central element of the baby-led approach is that babies are allowed to self-feed. Being in control of your own intake of food, and being able to stop eating when you are full is a really important step in developing healthy eating behaviours. There is a whole body of evidence for the importance of this for older children and we'll look at this in the next chapter. In short, mothers who adopt a responsive feeding style with their pre-school and school-aged children are more likely to have children who have healthy weight and eating behaviours. Understanding how baby-led weaning itself is different to responsive feeding is a really important research question. Baby-led weaning certainly encourages a responsive feeding approach, but is it this, or something about self-feeding or family foods in addition that might have a positive impact?

One of the most common responses I get when I discuss baby-led weaning in the media is that it is perfectly possible to spoon-feed responsively. I agree, and this is very important however you decide to introduce solid foods to your baby. Critics of baby-led weaning often say 'But it's obvious when my baby doesn't want any more, they turn their head away or refuse to open their mouth'. My response to this is to question the stage the baby is at when they clamp down or turn their head. Have they just got full? Or have they been quite full for a while, but you've carried on offering, so they've carried on eating? These small additional bites might not seem like much, but have an effect over time.

If a baby is self-feeding family foods it is likely that they eat at a slower pace than if they are being spoon-fed puréed foods that are easy to swallow. Self-feeding, especially at the start, is a skill that needs to develop. Chewing on food takes time. Joining in a family meal means you have more time to eat, rather than it being a rushed task before the main meal. All of this may lead to the mealtime taking longer. We know that adults who eat at a slower pace are less likely to be overweight. This is because they have time to register how much food has been eaten and when they feel full. The same may apply to babies who are self-feeding – they get to know the feeling of being full, and stop before they have overeaten. Again, this may only save a few calories at a time, but these all add up.

3. *Because they were more likely to have been breastfed*

At the moment, babies who are baby-led weaned are more likely to have been breastfed. Breastfeeding also helps to promote healthier weight and eating habits, so trying to untangle the two is important. Babies who were breastfed are less likely to be overweight as toddlers and children, possibly because they have been shown to eat more slowly (which helps you not to overeat) and to have better appetite control (so are less likely to eat more than they need).[12]

This may be because breastfed babies are more in control of their intake of milk than formula-fed babies are. Because you cannot see how much milk a breastfed baby has taken, so there is less temptation to encourage them to 'finish' a feed, as you might if there was milk left over in the bottle. Breastfed babies take in fewer calories at each feed right from the start of life, and feed more slowly. They also react to changing energy density in breastmilk, taking less when the milk is high in fat, and more when it is lower in fat. Formula milk is a uniform product that does not change with each feed, so babies do not need to adapt in the same way. Over time this might teach breastfed babies to control their appetite better. Breastfed babies are also less likely to be fussy eaters as toddlers and are more likely to accept a wider range of foods when they are introduced to solid foods.[13]

Any research that explores the impact of a baby-led approach on child eating behaviour and weight needs to examine whether the babies were breastfed and how this might affect any outcome.

4. Because they are self-feeding family foods

Babies who are following baby-led weaning are more likely to eat family foods. What is placed in front of them looks and tastes like the 'normal' version of the food. An apple looks like an apple, rather than a yellow purée. A pear looks like a pear, rather than a yellow purée. A chicken dinner looks like... you get the picture. Purées look very similar and may not be distinguishable by smell or even taste.

Why does this matter? It may have an impact on how we

learn about food. Firstly, food is more enjoyable when you are in control of it yourself. And young babies get a lot of fun and learning from food in addition to taste. What happens when I squish this? Does this rub in my hair? Look at mum's face when I drop this. This exploration is all part of the learning experience and is missing if you are spoon-fed foods of a similar consistency.

So baby-led weaning may encourage babies to learn more quickly about food. There is a theory of food learning that applies to adults that could be relevant for young babies too. As adults we learn over time what a food will make us feel like if we eat it. We know that a large roast dinner will make us feel full, whereas a fruit salad is unlikely to have the same effect. We match what the food looks and tastes like with how it made us feel.

It is possible that babies following a baby-led approach learn this more quickly. The shape in front of them that tastes, smells and fills them up a little is an apple. The bread has a different effect, as does this chicken. Spoon-feeding misses out this information, as all food looks and feels similar. Many shop-bought fruit purées have a rice or cornflour base for consistency and to add calories, and meal-type jars may contain water. This confuses the learning process.

5. Because of who chooses to baby-led wean

As with any research, it is important to know that it is the behaviour in question that leads to an outcome, rather than other factors. One of the issues with baby-led weaning research is that it follows the experiences of mothers who have chosen to follow a baby-led approach. It could be that these mothers are different in a number of ways to those who prefer a traditional approach. And these differences could be affecting outcomes.

Some studies have suggested that mothers who choose to follow baby-led weaning might be older, or have a higher level of education, which might enable them to provide a healthier diet later on. However, not all studies show this. What is interesting is that research suggests that mothers who choose to baby-led wean might have different attitudes to food, eating and weight than those who prefer a traditional approach.[14]

In particular, in one study I found that mothers who followed a baby-led approach were less likely to be restrained eaters (limiting their food intake, dieting a lot) than those following a traditional approach. Mothers of older children who are restrained eaters are more likely to have children who overeat, and as a consequence are more likely to be overweight. This is thought to be because a mother's concerns about weight gain extend to her child. She tries to limit what they eat, in terms of specific foods and how much. However, limiting a child too much can lead to them overeating when they get the opportunity. Restricting what children can eat breaks down their natural ability to regulate their own appetite. It is probable that if a mother is worried about her own weight and has concerns about her child becoming overweight, she would be uncomfortable with a baby-led approach that lets the baby decide when they are full.

Baby-led weaning has also been associated with lower maternal anxiety in general. This makes sense. If you are naturally more anxious, you can see why baby-led weaning might be more difficult. Are they eating enough? Is it OK for them to eat that food? Will they choke? A spoon-feeding approach might seem less anxiety provoking. In older children, maternal anxiety is associated with a more controlling feeding style, in terms of monitoring and keeping track of what a child eats, which discourages the child from regulating their own appetite.

6. Because of which babies can follow a baby-led approach

In theory, a baby-led approach should be suitable for most babies, although those with developmental delay, who cannot self-feed or who are failing to thrive may not be suited to it. However, it is possible that the characteristics of a baby might determine whether they start or continue baby-led weaning, and also affect later weight and eating behaviour.

For example, babies who are rated as having fussy temperaments are more likely to be fussy eaters when they are older. However, fussy babies are also more likely to be introduced to solid foods earlier, likely ruling out following baby-led weaning.[15] Babies who are perceived to be under- or overweight are also more likely to receive solid foods early, again meaning they are more likely to be spoon-fed.[16] If a baby is fussy, or even particularly hungry, the parent may be drawn to spoon-feeding in the belief that it will encourage them to 'just eat something' or 'get enough into them'. A lot more research needs to be done in this area.

Given these issues, the question of whether parents can ever really be randomised to follow the method or not is important. In the BLISS study, where mothers were randomised to either a baby-led or standard care approach, adherence to approach was monitored. At seven months, 64% of the baby-led group were classified as adherent to the principles of baby-led weaning. In comparison, 11% of the standard care group had adopted a baby-led approach. This suggests that it is not just as simple as suggesting that someone should follow baby-led weaning. Factors outside of this may influence choice to start or continue with it.

Getting support for the baby-led approach

Baby-led weaning can be a bit of a tricky area when it comes to seeking advice from health professionals. In some areas, practitioners are not allowed to give advice on baby-led weaning, while some don't feel they have the training and others might not want to give advice. This is because at present there are no Department of Health guidelines endorsing the baby-led approach (nor are there in other countries). This does not mean the method is unsafe, but simply that there is not enough of a scientific evidence base for guidelines to be drawn up.

Remember that there is no scientific evidence that spoon-feeding or purées are a safe or efficient way of introducing solid foods either. However, approaches that suggest a change to the accepted norm usually require an evidence base in order to be endorsed. The UK Department of Health does recommend finger foods from the start of weaning, so what is required is research that shows the efficacy of the baby-led approach in sufficiently supporting nutrient intake and growth. Given the small calorie requirements from solid foods in the early months, and the high incidence of obesity in the Western world, the approach also needs stronger evaluation as a preventative intervention.

The reluctance of some practitioners to support the baby-led approach is (perhaps ironically) supported by research. Mothers who follow baby-led weaning often report that their health visitor was unsure or unable to give advice on the approach, or sometimes said that they did not believe in following the method. Research with practitioners themselves often reveals a split. Many see potential benefits in the approach, believing it promotes responsive feeding, healthy weight gain and a wide intake of nutrients. However, many are also concerned that some babies might not eat enough, or that unsafe or inappropriate foods might be offered. In one Canadian study, less than half of health professionals noted that they were prepared to support their method in their own practice.[17]

The main infant feeding organisations in the UK have called for more research. Our research at Swansea that suggested a baby-led approach might decrease the risk of overweight attracted a lot of media attention. The media managed to spectacularly twist some of the messages of the research, but both the NHS and the Royal College of Paediatric and Child Health responded that more research was needed. The UNICEF Baby Friendly Initiative has also recently called for examination of the impact of the baby-led approach. The situation is the same in countries such as Australia, New Zealand, Canada and the US. So watch this space. For now, until we have more information, the most important message is that however you introduce solids to your baby, do it *responsively*.

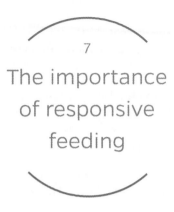

7

The importance of responsive feeding

What does 'responsive feeding' actually mean? And more importantly why does it matter? Responsive feeding can be defined as:

> *'a reciprocal relationship between an infant or child and his or her caregiver that is characterised by the child communicating feelings of hunger and satiety through verbal or nonverbal cues, followed by an immediate response from the caregiver. The response includes the provision of appropriate and nutritious food in a supportive manner, while maintaining an appropriate feeding environment'.*[1]

In other words – responsive feeding is about responding to cues of hunger and fullness in your baby or child and offering a wide range of healthy and appropriate foods in response to this. Responsive feeding is about more than just providing nutrients – it is about how the wider infant-parent relationship develops during feeds. It is about trust – both in terms of you trusting your baby that they will eat what they need, and your baby trusting that you will provide just that in a loving way. It is about meeting needs – giving enough food, but not pressurising a baby or child to eat more than they want. It is about offering a variety of tastes, but recognising that a child will not like them all. It is about providing food that is safe for the child. Responsiveness is a general parenting ethos rather than just about eating. And I believe it is just as important (if not more so) in developing positive, healthy eating behaviours as a nutritious diet.

Learning to recognise and understand your child's hunger and fullness cues is an intrinsic part of parenting. In babies these cues are different to those in toddlers, and they are different again in verbal children. Being able to recognise the first signs of satiety (fullness) is essential in not overfeeding children and supporting them to regulate their own appetite. Things like encouraging a baby to finish a bottle or eat just a few more spoons of a dish may feel as though they are coming from the right place, but in terms of supporting a child to regulate their own energy needs they are counterproductive.

We know that the most successful parenting comes when parents are responsive to their children. In infancy this includes responding promptly in appropriate ways that might include comfort, engagement, changing or feeding. Responsive parenting is associated with the best outcomes for children in terms of long-term emotional, social and educational wellbeing and even for wider health. When infants have their needs met they learn that they are loved and cared for and that someone will support them. They develop a first positive loving relationship, which acts as a template for further friendships and relationships. Feeding is central to this, because feeding is such a large part of a baby's life![2]

So it is not surprising that the World Health Organization views responsive feeding as one of the key criteria in how babies should be introduced to solid foods.

> *'Practice responsive feeding, applying the principles of psycho-social care. Specifically: a) feed infants directly and assist older children when they feed themselves, being sensitive to their hunger and satiety cues; b) feed slowly and patiently, and encourage children to eat, but do not force them; c) if children refuse many foods, experiment with different food combinations, tastes, textures and methods of encouragement; d) minimize distractions during meals if the child loses interest easily; e) remember that feeding times are periods of learning and love – talk to children during feeding, with eye to eye contact.'* [3]

Responsive feeding is important because it's not just about what a baby eats, but how they eat it. What their wider experience is like. How they feel about it. What they learn from it. And as we know, although feeding babies is about providing optimal nutrition, it's more than that – it's teaching them about fitting into our culture, relationships, emotions and more.

What's the evidence for responsive feeding?

Although you often hear about responsive feeding in relation to feeding babies both milk and solids, a lot of the wider literature actually comes from research with toddlers and school-aged children. These studies show that the best outcomes for encouraging children to develop positive eating behaviours (e.g. eating a wide range of different nutrients and not eating too much energy overall) come from feeding interactions that are responsive. Most of the research tends to look at how mothers interact with their children. Work is being done with fathers (and grandmothers and childcare workers, as they all play a role), but even when research is done with both parents, mothers seem to feel more responsibility and have more involvement with how and what their children eat. There seems to be more of a link between how she feels and how her child eats – which is a wider issue that research should address.[4]

What does responsive feeding mean for older children? It means offering a wide range of healthy options, but not being too 'controlling' about how much they eat. It involves a certain degree of trust and recognising that most children will eat when they are hungry. So yes, it involves serving healthy meals, encouraging children positively to try a bit if they refuse, but not putting too much pressure on them if they do not want to eat. It means filling the house with healthy snack options that children can eat if they are hungry. It means trying to praise the positives, such as trying new things, and not putting too much emphasis on the negatives. This can be difficult for a whole range of reasons (more below).

The best outcomes for children come from situations that encourage them to eat a range of nutrients – and this starts young. These include things like 'modelling' a healthy diet – eating a healthy diet yourself and hoping they will copy you. Parents who eat lots of fruit and vegetables themselves, and eat a wide, varied diet, are more likely to have children who eat in a similar way.[5] That's not to say you relinquish all control and oversight. Some control is a good thing. Providing them with lots of healthy snack options, but letting them choose what they want to eat from these, while limiting junk snack food options, is linked to children eating more nutrients and being a healthier weight.[6]

Responsive feeding works on the basis that children are born with an innate ability to control how much they eat. Indeed, most children are born with the ability to be 'satiety responsive', which means they generally only eat as much energy as they need and stop when they are full. People who are satiety responsive will be able to stop eating with food still on their plate and eat according to hunger rather than a set time on the clock or set portion sizes. They are the people who will say no to a cake offered if they are not hungry. This is the best way to be from a weight perspective, as people who are satiety responsive tend to be a healthy weight. They don't take in excess calories – and if they do, they naturally balance this with other smaller meals.

However, the problem with satiety responsiveness in our society is that it is based on an ability to follow your internal cues of hunger rather than what's going on around you in the world. Babies are born with this ability. However, our society often tries its best to dissuade us from being satiety responsive and by the time children reach school age they seem to have less ability to regulate how much they eat. Research with pre-school children shows that when you give them a high-energy starter they naturally eat less of a second main course. However, when they get a little older – at primary school age – they are not so good at doing this and tend to finish what is on their plate.[7]

So what happens? Ideas such as eating at set times rather than when you're hungry, cultural norms around clearing your plate and using food for reasons such as celebration rather than simply nutrition all encourage us to eat when we're not hungry. And our super-sized approach to food encourages us to eat even more – restaurant portion sizes are far bigger than they were even 20 years ago. All-you-can-eat buffets are popular. High fat, sweet-tasting foods are advertised wherever we look and constantly available. And our bodies are programmed to want them.

Parents can often struggle with encouraging and trusting their children to be satiety responsive. These are the very same small human beings who put beads up their noses to see what happens, don't understand about looking for traffic when crossing the road and like to see what happens when eggs drop on the floor. And yet we should trust them to know how much they want to eat? It's natural to worry about how much and what your child is eating, but sometimes the way parents deal with this can make the issue worse. If you worry about your child's diet, it is quite easy to step away from responsive feeding and become more controlling over what they eat. However, this is unfortunately where it can all go wrong.

There are two main non-responsive behaviours that have been identified that might have a detrimental effect upon how children eat and as a consequence how much they weigh. The first of these is 'restriction', which usually means trying to stop children eating larger portions, eating so frequently or eating particular foods. Foods tend to be those parents see as 'unhealthy' e.g. high in fat, energy or sugar rather than salads, although some parents will want to restrict overall energy intake. Research in this area often asks parents questions such as 'How much do you agree with statements such as: "I have to make sure my child does not eat too much of her favourite foods" or "I intentionally keep some foods out of my child's reach"?'

In theory, a bit of restriction sounds sensible, doesn't it? It is within certain boundaries, but only to some extent. The problem with restriction comes from that age-old concept of the forbidden fruit (or cake). The more you try not to have something, the more desirable it becomes. It's like when you go on a diet and can't stop thinking about all the foods you can no longer eat, even ones you never really wanted in the first place. What happens eventually? You end up breaking your diet and eating all the cake.

Research with parents shows that they often think restriction is a good idea. They think that by not exposing children to high-energy foods, their children will not want to eat them. But in experimental settings researchers have shown that telling children foods are forbidden or to be rationed actually increases how much they want them and how much they will then eat of them when allowed to. This even works when children rate two different snacks as similar in taste, but are then told they can only have a little of one. Suddenly that snack becomes more appealing![8] The more that parents report restricting, the more their children want to eat the restricted snacks. Parents who report very high levels of restriction have children who report wanting forbidden foods the most.[9]

The next step is looking at how much children will eat if allowed to, even if they are not hungry. Researchers often use a task called 'eating in the absence of hunger' to measure how much children will over eat a certain food if allowed to. Children are given a normal lunchtime meal and allowed to eat until they are full. They then are given another novel and attractive task to do – usually playing with new toys or in a new playroom or playground. While doing the task they are offered snack foods or told that there are snacks on the table for them to eat. Most children, even if they can control their own appetite, will try a snack or two. However, children who are particularly prone to eating in the absence of hunger will eat far more of these palatable snacks. Now guess which children eat more? Yes – the ones whose parents report restricting these snacks the most.

There also appears to be an increased impact when children know that they are not allowed these foods. Researchers find that the children of parents who report high levels of restriction eat far more when given free access to snack foods if the mother is not there compared to when she is.[10] Children essentially learn to eat in secret when they sense they are now allowed these certain foods.

The same phenomenon is seen even if children are not filled up with lunch. Very simply, if offered a meal with lots of palatable foods in it, children whose parents report restricting most will eat more than those who have parents who are more responsive. In real life, the party buffet often mimics this experiment – the children who are piling their plates high with food rather than just taking a few things are more likely to have parents who try and restrict food (or perhaps have particularly ferocious siblings who steal all the nice snacks at home).

One problem with restriction is that at first it seems to work. Particularly with a first-born child, restriction will work until a certain age. Toddlers and pre-school children do not have much control over their diets. They can't sneak foods from high cupboards, or take themselves off to the corner shop to buy a family-sized pack of cakes, so if parents want to restrict these foods they can and it works. Parents who report higher levels of restriction for their toddler have toddlers who eat less of those foods and are less likely to be overweight.[11]

However, you cannot keep children in a protective bubble forever. Eventually they will see adverts. They will go to school or parties and see their friends have snacks. They will have pocket money to spend in the shop – and be able to walk there without you. They will eventually eat these foods and most likely enjoy them and potentially eat as much of them as they possibly can, particularly if it is novel or restricted. You can see how parents who use lots of restriction are at greater risk of having a child who is overweight. But not every child of restrictive parents will be overweight, as weight is affected by lots of different factors, including genetics.

It's important to look critically at the relationship between restriction and being overweight, because what comes first? If you have a child who has a tendency to be overweight, it is only natural to try and restrict how many extra calories they consume. So any study that looks at a snapshot of weight and restriction might be drawing the wrong conclusion. However, longitudinal work in this area has tracked child weight and how parents interact with their child and found that although parents of children who are overweight are more likely to try and restrict, the restriction itself does have a negative impact. The more parents restricted, the more children ate when given free access and the more weight they put on.[12]

I want to emphasise here that all this isn't as simple as it sounds. If you're struggling with a child who is overweight, it's not the best advice to simply say 'don't restrict anything'! Research suggests that the best solution is to offer a wide range of healthy food options, with limited snacks. Cutting them out altogether just increases the longing. And the importance of genetics should not be ignored. Some children are programmed to put on weight more easily. Specific genes (and patterns of genes) have been shown to increase the risk that a child will struggle with overeating. Just because your child is drawn to overeating doesn't mean that you as a parent have done something 'wrong', just that your child is more susceptible to overeating. But minimising the impact is important.

A second common non-responsive behaviour is pressurising children to eat. Pressure to eat usually occurs during a meal and often for nutrient-dense foods, such as fruit and vegetables, which children might not be bothered about, but parents really want them to eat. Alternatively, the child may be encouraged to eat more of a meal even though they say they are full. Researchers tend to ask parents how much they agree with statements such as 'If I did not guide or regulate my child's eating she would eat less than she should' and 'My child should always eat all the food on the plate'.

The reasons for pressure to eat can vary. Some parents believe it will help their child to eat more nutrients or even like that food more. Some worry about their child's weight and growth. Pressure to eat can also be affected by the wider context – if you are on a low income and worried about food bills, pressurising a child to finish all the food on the plate even if they're full might feel like a necessity.

There is a difference between encouraging a child to try new things and to eat nutrient-dense foods and pressurising them. Offering new tastes, especially when you model eating them, and encouraging children to try a bit is a positive step. Prompting a child to focus on their meal rather than getting distracted, or reminding them to eat a little more now because you know they'll start demanding snacks three minutes after the food is in the dog's bowl is common sense. However, this can be a slippery slope to more negative behaviour – pressurising a child to eat when they are really not hungry or dislike a food.

Does pressure to eat encourage a child to like a food? Again this is very context-dependent. Offering a new food, enjoying it yourself and suggesting your child tries it, but being relaxed and moving on if they don't is great. Making your child eat a food they dislike… as it gets colder and colder… well, you probably have your own memories of what that's like. And a list of foods you still never try or eat as an adult. Research has shown that adults who dislike certain foods recall being made to eat them as a child.[13]

The research evidence shows a link between pressurising a

child to eat and fussy eating. Of course, if a child is very fussy it is only natural to worry that they are not getting sufficient nutrients and want to encourage them to eat more. Or to feel that your role as a parent is to make them eat it. And to some extent this explains the link, but it is not the full story.

Research from experimental settings shows that pressurising a child to eat a food decreases how much they like it, even if they didn't particularly dislike it in the first place. In one study children were asked to taste a soup and rate how much they liked it. When they were pressured to eat the whole bowl, their rating of it dropped.[14] Likewise, in 'real life', the more parents pressure their children to eat a certain food, the less they actually end up liking it and eating it. This could be due to attaching negative connotations to the food, such as 'I'm full, I don't want to eat this' or 'I don't like that food', or it could just be simple stubbornness! Who wants to eat something when they're full?

Often parents resort to bribes to try and get children to eat disliked foods. This isn't a great idea for a number of reasons, but importantly, in terms of getting children to actually like foods, it doesn't work. In one experiment, rewarding a child to eat more of a certain food increased how much they ate of that food, but decreased how much they liked it.[15]

Not all children will refuse to eat a food when pressured. Some will do as they're told and eat more than they need, potentially more so if they are at a genetic risk of overeating. The issue with this is that you risk breaking down your child's natural ability to self-regulate intake. This is unlikely to be such a problem if you are pressurising them to eat nutrient-dense but low-energy vegetables, but when parents think children should eat more than they are, or follow social customs not to waste food or finish everything on the plate, this can lead to more calories than needed being consumed.

In the West we seem to have a strange relationship with clean plates. How many people can recall as a child being told to finish everything on their plate as food musn't be wasted or it was rude not to? A common saying when I was a child was 'think of the starving children in Africa' – the strange suggestion that because others did not have enough food you must overeat. For some who are worried about money, this is more of a concern, but for those who do not need to worry so much about where the next meal is coming from this behaviour is bizarre if you think about it. Why encourage a child to eat too much? Why is continuing to eat when you are full a compliment? Why would you want a guest to make themselves uncomfortable when surely the point of serving them a meal was to offer them an enjoyable experience? These behaviours become ingrained – I speak to many adults who still worry about leaving things on the plate as they were encouraged to clear it as a child. Some older adults will hold memories from wartime when food was rationed and plate-clearing was important. That they are still conditioned to do it shows the strength of the behaviour.

And it is this conditioning that is the issue. The plate does not know how many calories you need or how big a breakfast you ate. And plate sizes are not uniform. People who show the best satiety responsiveness – and therefore usually the best energy regulation – are those who listen to internal rather than external signals. Eating because of what's on a plate or what someone else wants you to do is nonsensical. And the same applies to children. Now of course for some children a little encouragement to eat, as mentioned above, is needed, but the words are important – positive encouragement to eat a healthy amount is a good thing. Pressurising a child when they clearly do not want to eat is not.[16]

In terms of pressure to eat and weight the research is

not always conclusive, often because studies look at average weights or because pressure to eat can lead to either refusal or overeating. Generally, the more maternal pressure to eat, the lower the weight of the child. Again, the direction of this relationship is important. Does picky eating lead to low weight and therefore pressure to eat? Or does pressure to eat lead to picky eating and therefore slow weight gain? The evidence suggests both. Naturally, mothers who have a child who is underweight want to encourage them to eat more.[17] However, in longitudinal studies, pressure to eat increases the chances a child will have slower weight gain.[18]

What about using food to shape behaviour?

In an ideal world food should be about nutrition. We would eat the right nutrients and energy we needed when we needed it. However, we are far more complex than that and often eat or use food for reasons other than hunger. This isn't inherently wrong – after all, food is a large part of our culture and nobody would want to say you should ban all birthday cakes or family meal celebrations just because those nutrients aren't the right ones. As great as broccoli is, it doesn't really symbolise celebration!

The issue of food and celebration becomes more complicated when food is frequently used in non-nutritive ways. I think many of us are guilty of it at some point. 'You're not having pudding unless you finish your dinner' 'Eat those carrots or you can't have your ice cream' 'Be a good boy or you won't have any chocolate' 'If you tidy up your toys we'll get an ice cream at the park' 'Oh no, you've fallen over, will this chocolate make you feel better?' Or perhaps you're having a bad day and want to entertain the children easily. Harmless and a normal parenting tool? Maybe, but this sort of thing can cause problems.

There are two main ways we use food to shape behaviour. The first is using preferred foods (that are usually high in energy or sugar) as a bribe or reward for eating less preferred foods. Often this seems to work – the child reluctant to eat their main course suddenly finishes it in order to have the ice cream. But what does this teach them? To overeat when not hungry? That the main, nutrient-dense course is something to be endured to get to the treat? That the ice cream is something really special? Similarly, bribing a child with a treat to eat a disliked food may lead to the child thinking 'just how bad must that food be if mum is bribing me to eat it?' Bribing might get a child to eat a food, but it doesn't increase their liking of it.

The other issue is the long-term impact of all of this. Children and their diets are not under your control for very long. They start eating at school. They prepare their own meals. They somehow really quickly become adults and go out into the world. Will they still eat the foods they were bribed to eat as children, or will they skip straight to the prize, simply because they now can? Are you going to be ringing your 20-year-old daughter at university and telling her she can only eat the ice cream if she eats some vegetables?

A second issue can be using preferred foods outside of meal times to tackle behaviour. Favourite foods suddenly become not about mealtimes, but linked to making bad emotions better, as a suitable reward for doing mundane tasks, a symbol of praise when you achieve something... or a punishment if you're not allowed it. What does that teach children about food? And about eating in general? Fast forward to adulthood… you've broken up with a partner/had a particularly bad day with the children/ missed out on a promotion… how do you make yourself feel better? Many adults who comfort eat can remember being comforted with food as a child and it is a natural link. Parents who themselves comfort eat can be particularly prone to doing this with their children.

Children who are bribed regularly with food, either to reward their behaviour or to comfort their emotions, are at greater risk of overeating when they are not hungry and as a consequence at increased risk of becoming overweight.[19]

I'm worried about my child inheriting my weight problem

One of the biggest concerns that parents have for their children when it comes to nutrition is them becoming overweight. This is particularly true for mothers who have weight or body image issues when thinking about their daughters. Unfortunately, some of the ways that they handle this can actually exacerbate their children's risk of overweight.

Sometimes mothers who worry about their own weight have concerns for their daughters even if they are a healthy weight. Mothers with their own weight concerns are more likely to restrict certain foods in their daughter's diet, while pressurising them to eat nutrient-dense foods.[20] Likewise, mothers who themselves diet a lot are more likely to try and restrict their daughter's intake of snack foods.[21] Unfortunately this restriction can actually lead to an increased risk of their daughter eating in the absence of hunger.[22]

Children also are more aware of what you are really doing and feeling than you think they are. Research has shown that when mothers are emotional eaters, children are more likely to become so, even when the mother thinks she is not modelling this to them.[23]

Overall, a mother with poor body image and a restrictive eating style may be greatly concerned that her children will become overweight. Through restricting their intake of food she may believe she is doing her best for them, but in fact may be placing the child at greater risk of overweight.

How does this link with feeding babies?

Although a lot of the research discussed above has been done with older children, the lessons learned are transferable to feeding younger babies. Babies are typically born with a good ability to self-regulate, but it is important that they are fed responsively during infancy to maintain this ability. Even very early experiences can start to break this ability down.

Responsive feeding from birth is critical in helping to support babies to maintain their ability to regulate appetite, whether a baby is being fed from the breast or a bottle. Breastfed babies often take in less milk than formula-fed babies per feed.[24] One reason for this difference is that breastfed babies are more likely to be fed responsively than babies who are fed from a bottle. There are a number of reasons for this.

Firstly, it is more difficult to get milk 'out of' a breast. The baby has to actively latch on and stimulate the breast to make milk. It is not just a simple suck action, but one involving the tongue and jaw. Once the baby stops making the effort, the milk flow stops. A bottle-feeding baby is helped by gravity to get the milk out. This can mean that even when parents don't intend it, the baby might consume a little more at each feed before stopping.

Some parents encourage babies to try and 'finish off' bottles and my research showed that for some this was a desirable aspect of bottle-feeding. One study showed that when babies were encouraged to take more milk from a bottle, rather than stopping at the first sign the baby had enough, they took on average 10% more per feed.[25] Over time those small amounts add up. This may partly explain why formula-fed babies start taking in more calories from very early on.

Breastfeeding mothers are also more likely to feed their baby responsively in terms of timing, partly because feeding responsively is so important to building milk supply, and partly because it's difficult to encourage a baby to breastfeed for longer if they don't want to. Feeding little and often is really important however a baby is being fed, as babies are designed to feed frequently rather than having 'bigger' meals. Babies who have larger, less frequent feeds are more likely to become overweight.[26]

Breastfeeding can also help parents to be more responsive because to some extent you have to trust the baby to get what they need. Whereas a bottle has indicators on the side so you can see how much has been consumed, unless you get into weighing babies before and after feeds (and even that is unreliable) you are never going to know the exact amount a breastfed baby has consumed. Wet and dirty nappies, being alert and not looking dehydrated are good signs a baby is getting enough milk, but you still have to trust in a way you don't with a bottle. Research has shown that mothers who breastfeed go on to be more responsive at all later stages – introducing solids, and feeding toddlers and older children.[27]

My own research shows that responsive feeding during milk feeding is important for encouraging babies to be satiety responsive toddlers. We found that babies who were breastfed had better satiety responsiveness as toddlers, probably because they were more likely to be fed more responsively as babies.[28] Babies who exclusively breastfeed in the early months are also far less likely to finish large bottles of milk as older babies, suggesting they are self-regulating. Only 27% of exclusively breastfed babies finished bottles/cups of milk, compared to 68% who were only bottle fed.[29]

Parents are often surprised by how often a baby will feed if allowed to feed responsively. Breastfed babies naturally feed more often than formula-fed babies. Formula feeding has become so common in the UK that most parents have experience of bottle-feeding, compared to less than 1%

of parents who will exclusively breastfeed for six months. Breastfed babies feed on average every two hours compared to around every three hours for formula-fed babies.[30] Or at least they do in the West, where we tend to be more separate from our babies. In cultures where babies are typically held in a sling all day and co-sleep at night babies will often feed several times per hour for a few minutes at a time.[31]

Why do babies breastfeed more often than if they had formula? Mainly because breastmilk is digested more quickly. It is low in fat and protein, but high in carbohydrates and lactose, meaning that babies need to feed often. It is thought this might be an evolutionary survival mechanism, preventing mothers from leaving their vulnerable babies alone for too long. Breastfed babies also tend not to feed to a set pattern – they might have longer and shorter feeds, cluster feed or have growth spurts and seem to feed endlessly.

Breastfed babies also feed more slowly, drinking on average 8ml per minute compared to 28.5ml for formula-fed babies[32] and they tend to spend more time in sucking pauses than formula-fed babies.[33] Really they feed more like we eat and drink as adults – when we are hungry or thirsty, rather than at a set time. This might seem inconvenient or even anxiety-inducing for mothers, but it is, if you take a step back, just about feeding responsively to hunger.

Why don't babies breastfeed in a set pattern? Apart from the fact that adults don't eat in a set pattern, breastmilk isn't a uniform product. It changes over the course of a day and feeds, particularly in terms of fat and calorie content, therefore affecting when a baby will next be hungry. In warmer weather it can be less energy dense, encouraging babies to feed more. The fat content is lower at the start of a feed than at the end, and is higher at night.[34] Breastmilk constantly changes – and this is good, because it allows babies to experiment with their intake and 'hone' their satiety responsiveness.

Breastfed babies don't take set volumes at each feed and different babies feed for different lengths of time depending on the energy density of their mothers' milk. Although milk doesn't differ hugely between mothers, some produce milk that is higher in fat – and as a consequence their babies tend to have shorter feeds. Formula-fed babies do tend to drink the set feed they are given, meaning their feeding may be more predictable.[35]

Having said this, there is no reason why bottle-fed babies cannot be fed in a similar way, and responsive paced bottle feeding is a really important idea. Smaller feeds can be given carefully until the baby shows any sign of satiety and then stopped regardless of how much is in the bottle.

Responsive breastfeeding is also important for helping to build milk supply. Breastfeeding works on a demand and supply basis: the more the baby feeds, the more milk is produced. Removing breastmilk from the breast signals for more to be made – and the more the baby feeds, the more prolactin is produced (a hormone critical to good milk supply). Trying to feed to a routine by reducing the number of breastfeeds a baby has, or limiting time at the breast can reduce the amount of milk a mother produces, as the body thinks it is not needed. This can naturally lead to anxiety that the mother can't produce enough breastmilk – a worry that is often addressed by giving formula 'top-ups'. These end up further decreasing supply because the baby is not feeding at the breast.

When babies are breastfed responsively from birth, mature milk 'comes in' more quickly,[36] babies are more likely to get back to their birth weight quicker[37] and mums end up with a far better milk supply – most likely because babies have been shown to take in a third more milk than if they are fed less frequently.[38] Unsurprisingly, responsive breastfeeding is linked to exclusively breastfeeding for much longer.

What about milk feeding during solids?

A responsive feeding style remains important as babies are introduced to solid foods. If we remember how much solid food a baby needs at the start of weaning, it is a relatively small amount. The focus should be on giving milk feeds (responsively!) with some additional tastes and textures of solid food.

It is all too easy to start worrying about how much a baby is getting, and whether they are consuming the right nutrients, but hopefully the charts at the beginning of the book will show you how little babies really need. If a baby is going through a fussy stage, the focus should be on continuing to give tastes while maintaining milk supply, with additional vitamin drops if you are worried about your baby not receiving enough micronutrients. Breast or formula milk will still supply the majority of calories, fat and protein that your baby needs to grow and develop.

Recognising hunger and satiety cues is really important when introducing babies to solid foods. They have a little more control than babies do during milk feeding – after all they will now be able to sit up and move their head from side to side, clamp their mouth shut with some force or throw a bowl to the floor in rage! However, it is important to understand what are early signs of hunger and satiety and what are later ones – not only for your baby's appetite development but for all your wellbeing (and carpets).

Watching your baby as they eat and going at a slow pace are important in making sure your baby doesn't eat more than they really want. People often say 'I know when my baby is full, they turn their head away'. Is this really an early sign of satiety or a late one? To me it's a late sign that comes when they really do not want any more and are very full – just how many 'extra bites' have they had? More subtle signs are when babies are slowing down in their eating. Try offering the baby the spoon close to their mouth rather than putting it in – do they open their mouth eagerly to eat it, or have they lost interest? Are they still swallowing food, or are they pushing it out? Watch their facial cues and body language. Being alert to these more subtle cues can help your baby stay in control.

Ellyn Satter has an excellent resource in which she talks about the 'division of responsibility in feeding' which aligns perfectly with responsive feeding and letting babies be satiety responsive. She talks about how during the period when babies are introduced to solids, parents have the responsibility to provide the 'what' (e.g. what foods and in what form), along with the 'when' and 'where', while babies are responsible for deciding whether to eat and how much. Alongside providing the right foods (and a variety of them) parents also have a responsibility to make eating times pleasant and model how to behave at family mealtimes.[40]

In terms of the impact of responsive feeding during the weaning period, relatively little research has been done. Our research found that a responsive feeding style during the period babies are introduced to solid foods was associated with better satiety responsiveness and lower picky eating in toddlers.

A responsive feeding style during weaning appears to help babies regulate their weight to find their 'right place'. In one study researchers observed mothers feeding their babies at six months old. When mothers were responsive in their feeding style, infants who had had slow weight-gain during the first six months gained significantly more weight during the next six months and vice versa, thus balancing their weight gain.

Conversely, when mothers showed high levels of controlling feeding practices, babies who had had slow weight gain continued to gain weight at a slower rate, and those with initial greater weight-gain further increased theirs.[41]

In one research study of mothers of babies aged 6–12 months, we explored responsive feeding interactions and concerns. Mothers who perceived their baby as being larger were already starting to use restrictive feeding practices even at six months old. Notably, mothers who were themselves concerned about their own weight, or who were on a diet, were more likely to be restrictive with their baby.[42]

So learn your baby's signs of hunger and satiety. Offer a range of healthy options, but don't pressurise or stringently monitor day-to-day intake. The bigger picture really matters. Protecting your baby's ability to regulate their own appetite, alongside fostering positive emotions around eating and exposure to a range of healthy tastes will set your baby on the right path to long-term healthy eating habits.

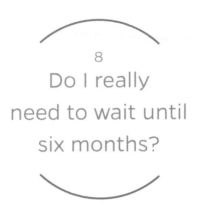

8

Do I really need to wait until six months?

So, the evidence for the when, what, how and why is logical, but that doesn't mean that decisions about when to introduce solids are straightforward. After all, the researchers aren't actually going to come and introduce solids to your baby for you. Furthermore, you will probably be surrounded by people (well meaning and otherwise) who think they should have a say in what goes on. Everyone's an expert in infant nutrition and they're going to tell you what they think. You might also still be concerned, despite all of this, that the guidelines aren't right for your baby. When parents reflect on why their baby was introduced to solid foods the answer is rarely 'because the guidelines said to do so at six months'. When we asked parents what their main reason for weaning was, only 7% mentioned the guidelines![1]

Most concerns around the timing of introducing solids stem from thinking that your baby needs solid foods before six months. The most common reasons given for introducing solid foods in the last UK Infant Feeding Survey were: a perception that the baby was no longer satisfied with milk feeds (52% of mothers), experience with a previous baby (30%), the baby was able to sit up and hold food in their hand (29%), advice from a health professional (27%) and that the baby was waking during the night (26%). It seems that the earlier solids are introduced, the more likely that reasons of hunger and not being satisfied with milk alone are given. Among mothers who had introduced solids by four months, 64% gave the reason that their baby was not satisfied with milk feeds alone.[2] These concerns are common and similar issues are reflected in research in many countries including the US, Canada, Australia, New Zealand and other European countries.

However, these concerns are not necessarily best addressed by introducing solid foods. Often, if you do try, you end up with the same problems and more mess and hassle!

My mother says she introduced me to solids at six weeks and I'm fine

This is always a difficult one as it can be tricky to seemingly defy her experience by doing something so different. However, we've seen that until the 1980s parents were advised to introduce solids at around three months, with many doing so sooner. The only reason the guidance has changed is that we have done more research and realised that it wasn't a great idea for babies to have solids so soon. She gave you solids when she thought was best, based on the advice of the time, and you are doing the same now.

However, our relationships with our mothers can make discussing such issues difficult, and perhaps a simple response such as 'this is what I'm doing with my baby' may work to calm things down. If you can, change the subject or ask for her advice about something else. But if deep down you're wondering whether she's right, there are a number of things to consider.

You may well be 'fine' as everyone is different. Research shows that earlier introduction of solids increases the risk of several illnesses, but it does not show that it causes these things in everyone. Health is rarely definitive. We all know someone who smoked 40 cigarettes a day, ate a terrible diet and had a fondness for whisky who lived to 106. Even if you have a 50% chance of experiencing an illness if you do something, you still have a 50% chance of not having it. All public health advice can do is tell people about the increased chances – and you make decisions based on that information.

The statistics are based on the risk of developing an illness across a whole population. Research looks at how many babies were introduced to solids at an earlier age and compares their illness levels to those who were given solids later. Any increase is then worked out as an increased probability of getting that illness. It is usually expressed as an 'odds ratio'; for example, your odds of getting a certain illness are 1.5 times higher if... However, it's not quite as simple as that as lots of other factors are involved. For some people the risk might be lower and for others, far higher. We know that some things are cumulative and factors including poverty, previous feeding experience, birth or pregnancy may all have an effect. One big thing that we know is important but is difficult to understand on an individual level (at least not without paying a lot of money) is genetics.

Everyone has a genetic risk of illness – for some this genetic risk will be higher, while for some it will be less. It's unlikely to be down to one individual gene, and more likely to be in the interplay between lots of different genes – making it even more difficult to test for. When we know that certain illnesses are increased when solids are introduced early, it is likely that the risk is higher for those with a genetic risk of that illness. Take autoimmune disorders for example. If you are in a family that has lots of autoimmune disorders, this might increase your awareness, but people can have illnesses that have a strong genetic component that are not seen in their immediate family. So really we only know the increased risk across the whole population. At present we don't understand enough about how genes and environment interact, but it is likely that if you have a genetic risk for an illness that is associated with an earlier introduction, then introducing solids early may trigger that illness more often than if you didn't have that genetic risk.

'Fine' is also subjective. It's often said that if you look at a class of school children or older adults, you cannot tell who was introduced to solids early and who was not. This is because there is not some dramatic, definitive event that happens if a baby has solid foods early. They don't turn bright green or grow an extra head. The differences are typically more subtle than that. As described previously, research has shown that babies introduced to solids earlier are at greater risk of certain illnesses, including digestive issues, infections and autoimmune disorders. Often we don't tell others when we have these conditions. Nor are these conditions caused by one event (early solids) – they can be triggered by lots of things or a combination of things.

Further, one of the main benefits of delaying solids is a decrease in gastrointestinal infections. Some studies show that this decrease only lasts until solids are introduced – so this might 'just' be a reduced risk of infection for three months in infancy. Gastrointestinal infections can be very serious for young babies – and even milder ones are not exactly fun. So although no one is turning green and growing another head, these small things do matter.

But my baby wakes up at night

A common belief is that if a baby is not sleeping through the night, introducing solids, or giving more of them just before bed, will help them to sleep. Around a quarter of mothers in the UK Infant Feeding Survey gave this reason for introducing solids, with around a third giving this reason if they introduced solids at 3–4 months. Unfortunately, this is a persistent myth. My own research shows that the amount of solids given does not affect sleep (and while we're on the subject, milk type does not affect sleep once the baby is past a few weeks old either – stopping breastfeeding will not help your baby to sleep).[3] Research has also shown that a bottle before bed doesn't work, nor does cereal before bed.[4]

There are also some risks in trying to 'fill a baby up' before bed. As adults we are unlikely to try and lie down and sleep right after a big meal because it is uncomfortable, and the same goes for babies. Overfeeding can mean that you are up more with a baby who is unsettled or in pain as they are simply too full, have wind or are constipated from the overload of solid foods. Trying to get them to eat when they're not hungry can also lead to them learning to overeat when food is offered, rather than simply eating when they're hungry.

It is normal for babies to wake up at night throughout the first year and beyond. The idea that babies should start to sleep through from a very early stage is nonsensical and research backs this up, showing how common it is for babies to wake at night. Depending on which research study you read, somewhere between 30 and 80% of babies aged 6–12 months still wake up at night, with the most common number of times to wake up being once or twice.[5] Waking in the night is also thought to be protective – sleeping too deeply may be associated with an increased risk of sudden infant death syndrome (SIDS), which is why the advice to give a dummy to babies is given – it stops them from sleeping too deeply.[6]

At this point I bet you are thinking about someone you know who has told you that waking up lots at night is linked to all sorts of terrible things. Yes, for older school-aged children, sleep problems can be linked to behavioural, academic and emotional issues.[7] But a baby waking up once or twice at night is not actually a sleep problem. It might feel like one to you, but it isn't for your baby. And there is no evidence to show that how a baby sleeps (or doesn't) will be its pattern for life. Even when toddlers are considered to have medical sleep issues, it doesn't predict their ability to sleep at six years old.[8] Fast forward a few years and you will be moaning at them for not getting out of bed before midday.

Also, babies wake up at night for reasons other than hunger. After all, adults wake up all the time at night and it's not because they need a snack. Babies may be cold, need a nappy changed, have come out of a sleep cycle, have been disturbed or simply want to be close to someone. As adults we wake for similar reasons, but are capable of getting ourselves back to sleep as we can sort out our own needs. Sometimes we may seek the comfort of a partner, who hopefully responds to your needs. Imagine waking from a particularly bad dream, wanting a hug and your partner completely ignoring you.

Often babies do wake up for a feed at night, but trying to replace this feed with solids during the day doesn't work. One reason for this is the simple equation of energy density. Solids can end up replacing milk, rather than being in addition to it. Filling a baby with carrot purée offers fewer calories and other nutrients than milk. So this will not solve the issue of a hungry baby. For a while they might want even more milk feeds. Feeding at night is also perfectly normal. In cultures where feeding at night is the norm, and parents don't try to restrict it, most babies feed around four times a night throughout the first year. Sometimes as babies get older they actually feed more at night as they were busy during the day.[9]

My research shows that most breastfed babies still have one or two night feeds at six months, and that this is completely unrelated to how much solid food they have in the day. Those who have a taste or two wake up as often as those who have several meals. My data does show that babies who are formula fed are less likely to have a feed at night… but they are no less likely to *wake* at night, meaning they still needed the same care and attention.[10] There are a number of possible explanations for this. Firstly, mothers who formula feed are more likely to track and measure the amount of milk a baby has, so they may feel that the baby has had enough during the day and try to get them back to sleep without a feed. It is very difficult to judge how much milk a breastfed baby has had, so perhaps mothers feed them back to sleep 'just in case'.

However, breastfeeding is a pretty handy tool at night. Whip out a breast, latch the baby on and they're probably sound asleep again in a few moments. So that baby may have had a night 'feed', but do we know how much they took in? Probably not enough to count as a meal to satisfy hunger – more likely the baby wanted the comfort of latching on to the breast. This fits with research that shows that although breastfed babies are fed more at night, mums who breastfeed actually get more sleep overall because they can get back to sleep so quickly, without needing to make a bottle.[11]

Babies often feed more at night when they are going through a growth spurt (or just before one). There is a huge growth spurt and developmental leap at around four and a half months old. This fits neatly with data showing how much babies wake up at night. A Swedish study that tracked how often babies fed at night found that the average number of night feeds at two weeks old was 2.2 feeds, reducing to 1.3

at 12 weeks before rising again to 1.8 at 20 weeks. At four months 48% fed once at night, 37% twice, 11% three times and 3% four times. However, this dropped back down to lower levels just after 20 weeks. Given that we are often told that solid foods are needed at around four or five months old, this begs a question. Are solids needed? Or was baby just having a growth spurt?[12]

Finally, sometimes babies do wake because they are thirsty rather than hungry. That's OK. Adults do too. Many of us sleep with a glass of water beside our bed. It's probably less acceptable to keep cake there (unless you're up feeding a baby, in which case it's totally fine). Why not afford babies the same comfort too? Milk, particularly if you're breastfeeding, isn't just about nutrition. Breastfeeding a baby back to sleep is completely normal human behaviour.

My baby is a big baby and needs something more

A common reason for introducing solid foods earlier than recommended is having a big baby. The rationale is that bigger babies have different calorie needs to smaller babies and need solid foods sooner. However, given the size of babies, this doesn't really make much sense. Firstly, the calorie needs of 'average' and large babies at around 4–6 months are really not that different. Babies and children between the ages of three months and three years need approximately 90–100 calories per kilogram of body weight per day. At about four months old, your average 50th percentile baby weights around 7.5kg, whereas a 98th percentile baby is closer to 9kg. This means that your larger baby will need only around 120 calories a day more than your average baby.

Looking at how they could get those extra calories, milk has far more calories and fat than most solid foods. Per 100ml, breastmilk has around 67 calories and 4g fat, and formula milk around 66 calories and 3.5g fat. Conversely, typical foods you might give to a baby under six months old would be fruit and vegetables. A 100g serving of vegetable purée has just 39 calories and 0.2g fat. Even 100g of baby porridge has only around 60 calories and 0.3g fat.

A baby's tummy is about the size of its fist. In countries where solids are introduced at four to six months, the recommended intake is 1–3 tablespoons of food, twice a day at most. A tablespoon represents about 15g of food. Even at the six tablespoons end of that advice, you'd only be giving around 35 extra calories a day. If you gave porridge it would be about 55 calories. If you introduce solids early because you want to give more calories, it's likely you'll end up actually giving less.

Getting food into a young baby who has a tongue reflex to push it out is going to be hard work. Even ignoring the health factors discussed earlier, if you feel your baby needs more calories, it is simpler and easier to give them more milk. To get that extra 100 calories, you are looking at around 15–20 minutes extra breastfeeding over the course of the day (roughly a baby will take around 150ml per 15 minutes, some quicker, some slower). Given that breastfed babies very naturally self-regulate their intake, this might mean an extra feed or slightly longer feeds. If you're formula feeding, this equates to around 150ml more formula (roughly two-thirds of an extra bottle). If you're worried about adding extra volume to a bottle, you can simply offer an extra feed, bringing feeds closer together.

I can't produce enough breastmilk for a big baby

Actually you most probably can, as long as you feed your baby responsively, whenever they want it. Your body will just increase its supply. This is one reason why many babies seem to go through a difficult phase at about four months when they feed very often – it's because they are building up the supply ready for a growth spurt. Many women exclusively breastfeed twins or even triplets, and historically wet nurses often fed up to six babies at once![13] As we've seen, the additional amount of milk needed is fairly small – about 100ml (about 15% more).

My baby's growth is slowing down

Many parents start to worry when they see that their baby's growth starts to slow down, as they approach six months old, but this is completely normal. The most rapid growth comes in the first month and then it starts to slow down. If we grew at the same rate we did in that first month…. we'd weigh several tonnes as adults! If you look at the growth charts in your baby's record book you will see that the line is steepest in the early months, before starting to taper into a curve from around 3–4 months. So it is normal for your baby's growth to slow down. It does not mean they are starving and desperately need food.

Babies with higher birth weights often slow their weight gain earlier than lower birth weight babies. They're just settling into their natural growth pattern, but this can often be misinterpreted as something being wrong. It's natural to feel a certain sense of pride when you get your baby weighed and see they have grown, and it can feel disconcerting when this starts to change. But it's normal – and even if it wasn't, the best response is to offer calorie-dense breast or formula milk, not solids.

My baby keeps looking at my food!

Yes, he does. He also looks at your face, but I'm guessing he doesn't want to eat you. Or he watches you use a knife or drive the car, but you're not going to let him do that yet. It's normal for babies to watch what we're doing and copy our movements

– opening and closing our mouths, picking things up and putting them in… it's how they learn to do things. They also get great enjoyment from copying – it's why they like games where you copy their movements or sounds. It helps them learn about the world and also strengthens the bond between you. But does this mean they are trying to frantically signal they want food?

It's unlikely your baby is asking for food in this way, primarily because they have no idea what eating food is actually like. They don't understand that putting food in your mouth means you chew and swallow it and feel full. Food to them comes from the breast or in a bottle. It tastes like milk. They may pick up other items and chew or gum them, but they don't eat them. Thinking that they really want a bit of the tasty meal you are eating is transferring your knowledge of food to them.

If my baby can eat food they will be more advanced

It is normal to be proud of things your baby does, but eating solid foods is a physical skill that develops when your baby is ready. It is not something you can teach them and it does not mean they are more advanced if they are ready earlier. There is absolutely no link between being ready to have solids and later achievement or wellbeing. There is no developmental benefit to early introduction. In fact, babies will probably get more enjoyment and learning from the process if they are allowed to go at their own pace when they are ready.

But I'm really excited to move on

Giving first foods to your baby is exciting. Choosing them, preparing them, watching their face as they eat it. The mess. It's all great fun for the first few times and then… well, I think at some point we all think back to just giving them milk and realise how simple that was. Once you've started it's hard to go back. And the younger you start the more complicated it is. Getting those cookbooks out and making tiny cubes of food… exciting at the start, less so when it's what feels like the millionth ice-tray-full in the freezer. Also, the earlier you start, the more mess and waste you'll have to put up with. Still sound exciting?

My baby has teeth
Some babies are born with teeth. This is not a reason to introduce solids early. Babies do not need teeth for chewing anyway.

Don't boys need solid foods earlier?
Boys are more likely to be introduced to solid foods early than girls, often because they are perceived to be bigger, or more hungry. Again, if a baby is bigger, they need more milk rather than solids. Boys do consume more milk and feed more often, but the difference is really only significant on a statistical rather than day-to-day level. It's not like boy babies feed every hour and girls only every three hours.[14]

Interestingly, or perhaps more worryingly, when we did research exploring why babies were given solid foods, while boys were being introduced early because of perceived hunger, we found girls were more likely to have solids in order to 'make them more settled'. Might this be because girl babies are more demanding than boy babies? Nope. Observations show that girls are actually more settled, sleep more and cry less than boys.[15] Is this gender stereotyping? There are lots of studies showing that adults interact differently with male and female babies – holding girls more gently, talking to them in a hushed voice and not bouncing them as much. The same is true of older children: contrast 'boys will be boys' allowing boys to

141

be more boisterous, with girls being expected to be quieter. In other work we found that parents are more likely to see female infants as manipulative and needing their behaviour shaping than male infants.[16] Given the belief that solids might improve sleep, parents may therefore be using solids to try and do this.

What about professional advice?

It would not be appropriate for me to question medical advice you are given for your individual baby. However, do consider who is giving the advice, what training they've had and their rationale for why solids are needed. Some professionals may still advise solids for spurious reasons such as sleep and weight gain when in fact babies are a perfectly healthy weight. Do not be afraid to ask why solids are being recommended and how they will help. Get a second opinion if this doesn't seem clear. If your baby has significant weight issues, allergies or severe reflux speak to your GP or a dietician about the best way forward.

We've looked at some of the reasons why you might think – or others might tell you – that your baby should be getting solid foods before six months. Usually these involve behaviours unrelated to food, and as a consequence food is unlikely to change them. Although it might not seem like it at the time, the period between when you first consider giving solids and them reaching six months old is really quite short. Hang on in there. It will pass and you will probably be grateful for the mess you avoided!

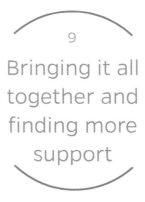

9

Bringing it all together and finding more support

So, we've reached the end of the book. But what should be the key take-away messages if you're introducing solids, helping someone else or just generally interested? I think the following 10 steps sum up what you really need to know.

1. Try to delay solids until six months. There is generally no benefit in starting any earlier and you reduce the risk of infections by delaying.

2. The first few months of solid foods are about tastes and textures, not amounts. Babies actually need very little and these foods should be the best possible choices.

3. Milk should still be a major part of the diet. You do not need follow-on formula, whatever the adverts might tell you, whether you're breast or bottle feeding.

4. Commercial baby foods are fine occasionally and can be convenient. However, they tend to be high in

sugar and lack the range of textures home-cooked food provides, so don't give them all the time.

5. Remember the baby food industry is there to sell products – the more you buy of their product the better for them and the worse for your pocket.

6. Whatever approach you take to introducing solids, remember the importance of responsive feeding.

7. Baby-led weaning makes a lot of sense because it promotes good choices such as delaying solids, family mealtimes and responsive feeding.

8. Foods are not magical. They will not help your baby sleep.

9. If a baby is hungry, or a 'big baby', the best choice is to give more breast or formula milk as it is energy dense. You can make enough breastmilk for your baby, but feeding frequently (responsively) is crucial.

10. Relax. It is likely your baby is getting enough.

Where to get more support and information

- The First Steps Nutrition Trust website contains a wealth of information about introducing solids, portion sizes and healthy eating in the early years **firststepsnutrition.org/newpages/Infants/first_year_of_life.html**

- The Ellyn Satter Institute explores the importance of introducing your baby to solid foods with a mission to help children be joyful with eating **ellynsatterinstitute.org**

- The Child Feeding Guide (and Feeding Kids UK social media pages), run by child feeding researchers, are a great source of advice, in particular for strategies for overcoming fussy eating **childfeedingguide.co.uk**

- Every parent should do a First Aid course and the Red Cross have a great video on saving a choking **babyredcross.org.uk/What-we-do/First-aid/Baby-and-Child-First-Aid/Choking-baby**

- The UNICEF UK Baby Friendly Initiative has a great leaflet on introducing solids **unicef.org.uk/babyfriendly/baby-friendly-resources/leaflets-and-posters/weaning-starting-solid-food**

- Start4Life also have lots of useful information **nhs.uk/start4life/first-foods**

- For baby-led weaning advice, start at **babyledweaning.com**

- For support in continuing to breastfeed the National Breastfeeding Helpline is run in collaboration with the Breastfeeding Network and the Association of Breastfeeding Mothers. Call 0300 100 0212 to speak to a trained volunteer. **nationalbreastfeedinghelpline.org.uk**

- For unbiased information about formula milks, the First Steps Nutrition website is invaluable **firststepsnutrition.org/newpages/Infant_Milks/infant_milks.html**

- KellyMom **kellymom.com**

- Analytical Armadillo blog: **analyticalarmadillo.co.uk**

- My own site: Breastfeeding Uncovered **breastfeedinguncovered.co.uk**

- For information about unscrupulous formula
  milk marketing, see Baby Milk Action's website
  babymilkaction.org

Further reading

My Child Won't Eat!: How to enjoy mealtimes without worry,
Carlos Gonzales, Pinter & Martin, 2012.

Complementary Feeding: Nutrition, Culture and Politics,
Gabrielle Palmer, Pinter & Martin, 2011.

*Inventing Baby Food: Taste, Health, and the Industrialization of
the American Diet*, Amy Bentley, University of California
Press, 2014.

Baby-led Weaning: Helping Your Baby to Love Good Food, Gill
Rapley and Tracy Murkett, Vermilion, 2008.

*Baby Self-Feeding: Solutions for Introducing Purées and Solids
to Create Lifelong, Healthy Eating Habits*, Nancy Ripton
and Melanie Potock, Fair Winds Press, 2016.

Milk Matters: Infant feeding and immune disorder, Maureen
Minchin, Milk Matters Pty Ltd, 2015

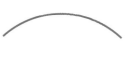

References

Chapter 1

1. Konner, M., & Worthman, C. (1980). Nursing frequency, gonadal function, and birth spacing among !Kung hunter-gatherers. *Science*, 207(4432), 788-791.
2. Castilho, S.D., & Barros Filho, A.D.A. (2010). The history of infant nutrition. *Jornal de pediatria*, 86(3), 179-188.
3. Bentley, A. (2014). *Inventing Baby Food: Taste, Health, and the Industrialization of the American Diet* (Vol. 51). Univ of California Press.
4. United States Children's Bureau (1929) Infant Care guidance ia802605.us.archive. org/19/items/infantcare00unit/infantcare00unit.pdf
5. Palmer, G. (2011). *Complementary feeding: nutrition, culture and politics*. Pinter & Martin.
6. Truby King, M. (1941). *Mothercraft*. Whitcombe and Tombs Ltd, Sydney.
7. Sackette, W. (1953) *Bringing up babies: a family doctor's practical approach to child care*. Harper & Row.
8. Fildes, V.A. (1986). *Breasts, bottles and babies: a history of infant feeding*.
9. Oates, R.K. (1973). Infant-feeding practices. *BMJ*, 2(5869), 762.
10. Wilkinson, P.W., & Davies, D.P. (1978). When and why are babies weaned? *BMJ*, 1(6128), 1682-1683.
11. World Health Organization (1981) International Code of Marketing of Breast-Milk Substitutes www.who.int/nutrition/publications/code_english.pdf
12. McAndrew, F., Thompson, J., Fellows, L., Large, A., Speed, M., & Renfrew, M.J. (2012). *Infant Feeding Survey 2010*. Health and Social Care Information Centre.

Chapter 2

1. www.who.int/nutrition/topics/complementary_feeding/en/
2. www.unicef.org.uk/babyfriendly/baby-friendly-resources/leaflets-and-posters/ weaning-starting-solid-food/
3. www.aap.org/en-us/advocacy-and-policy/aap-health-initiatives/HALF-

Implementation-Guide/Age-Specific-Content/pages/infant-food-and-feeding.aspx

4. www.espghan.org/guidelines/nutrition/

5. www.health.gov.au/internet/publications/publishing.nsf/Content/gug-director-toc~gug-solids

6. World Health Organization (2003) *Global Strategy for Infant and Young Child Feeding*.

7. Kramer, M.S., & Kakuma, R. (2002). Optimal duration of exclusive breastfeeding (Review). *Cochrane database of systematic reviews*, 1, 11-12.

8. Lanigan, J.A., Bishop, J.A., Kimber, A.C., & Morgan, J. (2001). Systematic review concerning the age of introduction of complementary foods to the healthy full-term infant. *European Journal of Clinical Nutrition*, 55(5), 309.

9. Moorcroft, K.E., Marshall, J.L., & McCormick, F.M. (2011). Association between timing of introducing solid foods and obesity in infancy and childhood: a systematic review. *Maternal & Child Nutrition*, 7(1), 3-26.

10. Carter, C. A., & Frischmeyer-Guerrerio, P. A. (2018). The genetics of food allergy. Current allergy and asthma reports, 18(1), 2.

11. Nwaru, B.I., Hickstein, L., Panesar, S.S., Roberts, G., Muraro, A., & Sheikh, A. (2014). Prevalence of common food allergies in Europe: a systematic review and meta-analysis. *Allergy*, 69(8), 992-1007.

12. Poole, J. A., Barriga, K., Leung, D. Y., Hoffman, M., Eisenbarth, G. S., Rewers, M., & Norris, J. M. (2006). Timing of initial exposure to cereal grains and the risk of wheat allergy. Pediatrics, 117(6), 2175-2182.

13. Kull, I., Bergström, A., Lilja, G., Pershagen, G., & Wickman, M. (2006). Fish consumption during the first year of life and development of allergic diseases during childhood. Allergy, 61(8), 1009-1015.

14. Shreffler, W. G., & Radano, M. (2011). Food allergy and complementary feeding. In *Early Nutrition: Impact on Short-and Long-Term Health* (Vol.68, pp.141-152). Karger Publishers.

15. Du Toit, G., Roberts, G., Sayre, P.H., Plaut, M., Bahnson, H.T., Mitchell, H., ... & Lack, G. (2013). Identifying infants at high risk of peanut allergy: the Learning Early About Peanut Allergy (LEAP) screening study. *Journal of Allergy and Clinical Immunology*, 131(1), 135-143.

16. Perkin, M.R., Logan, K., Marrs, T., Radulovic, S., Craven, J., Flohr, C., ... & EAT Study Team. (2016). Enquiring About Tolerance (EAT) study: feasibility of an early allergenic food introduction regimen. *Journal of Allergy and Clinical Immunology*, 137(5), 1477-1486.

17. Zeiger, R.S., & Heller, S. (1995). The development and prediction of atopy in high-risk children: follow-up at age seven years in a prospective randomized study of combined maternal and infant food allergen avoidance. *Journal of Allergy and Clinical Immunology*, 95(6), 1179-1190.

18. Zeiger, R.S., Heller, S., Mellon, M.H., Forsythe, A.B., O'Connor, R.D., Hamburger, R.N., & Schatz, M. (1989). Effect of combined maternal and infant food-allergen avoidance on development of atopy in early infancy: a randomized study. *Journal of Allergy and Clinical Immunology*, 84(1), 72-89.

18. Schoetzau, A., Filipiak-Pittroff, B., Franke, K., Koletzko, S., Von Berg, A., Gruebl, A., ... & Wichmann, H. (2002). Effect of exclusive breast-feeding and early solid food avoidance on the incidence of atopic dermatitis in high-risk infants at 1 year of age. *Pediatric Allergy and Immunology*, 13(4), 234-242.

20. Grimshaw, K.E., Maskell, J., Oliver, E.M., Morris, R.C., Foote, K.D., Mills, E.C., ... & Margetts, B.M. (2013). Introduction of complementary foods and the relationship to food allergy. *Pediatrics*, 132(6), e1529-e1538.

21. Akobeng, A.K., Ramanan, A.V., Buchan, I., & Heller, R.F. (2006). Effect of breast feeding on risk of coeliac disease: a systematic review and meta-analysis of observational studies. *Archives of Disease in Childhood*, 91(1), 39-43.

22. Norris, J.M., Barriga, K., Hoffenberg, E.J., Taki, I., Miao, D., Haas, J.E., ... & Rewers, M. (2005). Risk of celiac disease autoimmunity and timing of gluten introduction in the diet of infants at increased risk of disease. *JAMA*, 293(19), 2343-2351.

23. Michaelsen, K.F., Weaver, L., Branca, F., & Robertson, A. (2000). *Feeding and Nutrition of Infants and Young Children: Guidelines for the WHO European Region, with Emphasis*

on the Former Soviet Countries. WHO Regional Publications, European Series, No.87.

24. Dewey, K.G., Cohen, R.J., Brown, K.H., & Rivera, L.L. (2001). Effects of exclusive breastfeeding for four versus six months on maternal nutritional status and infant motor development: results of two randomized trials in Honduras. *The Journal of Nutrition,* 131(2), 262-267.

25. Hollis, B.W., Wagner, C.L., Howard, C.R., Ebeling, M., Shary, J.R., Smith, P.G., ... & Hulsey, T.C. (2015). Maternal versus infant vitamin D supplementation during lactation: a randomized controlled trial. *Pediatrics,* 136(4), 625-634.

26. Dewey, K.G. (2001). Nutrition, growth, and complementary feeding of the breastfed infant. *Pediatric Clinics of North America,* 48(1), 87-104.

Chapter 3

1. Rapley, G. (2011). Baby-led weaning: transitioning to solid foods at the baby's own pace. *Community Practitioner,* 84(6), 20.

2. Naylor, A.J., & Morrow, A.L. (2001). *Developmental Readiness of Normal Full Term Infants To Progress from Exclusive Breastfeeding to the Introduction of Complementary Foods: Reviews of the Relevant Literature Concerning Infant Immunologic, Gastrointestinal, Oral Motor and Maternal Reproductive and Lactational Development.*

3. Illingworth, R.S., & Lister, J. (1964). The critical or sensitive period, with special reference to certain feeding problems in infants and children. *The Journal of Pediatrics,* 65(6), 839-848.

4. Northstone, K., Emmett, P., & Nethersole, F. (2001). The effect of age of introduction to lumpy solids on foods eaten and reported feeding difficulties at 6 and 15 months. *Journal of Human Nutrition and Dietetics,* 14(1), 43-54.

5. Brown, A., & Lee, M.D. (2015). Early influences on child satiety-responsiveness: the role of weaning style. *Pediatric Obesity,* 10(1), 57-66.

6. Rapley, G. (2015). Baby-led weaning: The theory and evidence behind the approach. *Journal of Health Visiting,* 3(3), 144-151.

7. Mennella, J.A., & Trabulsi, J.C. (2012). Complementary foods and flavor experiences: setting the foundation. *Annals of Nutrition and Metabolism,* 60(Suppl. 2), 40-50.

Chapter 4

1. Michaelsen, K.F., Weaver, L., Branca, F., & Robertson, A. (2000). *Feeding and Nutrition of Infants and Young Children: Guidelines for the WHO European Region, with Emphasis on the Former Soviet Countries.* WHO Regional Publications, European Series, No.87.

2. www.who.int/nutrition/topics/complementary_feeding/en/

3. www.unicef.org.uk/babyfriendly/baby-friendly-resources/leaflets-and-posters/weaning-starting-solid-food/

4. McAndrew, F., Thompson, J., Fellows, L., Large, A., Speed, M., & Renfrew, M. J. (2012). *Infant Feeding Survey 2010.* Health and Social Care Information Centre.

5. Friel, J.K., Hanning, R.M., Isaak, C.A., Prowse, D., & Miller, A.C. (2010). Canadian infants' nutrient intakes from complementary foods during the first year of life. *BMC Pediatrics,* 10(1), 43.

6. Koletzko, B., von Kries, R., Closa, R., Escribano, J., Scaglioni, S., Giovannini, M., ... & Sengier, A. (2009). Lower protein in infant formula is associated with lower weight up to age 2y: a randomized clinical trial. *The American Journal of Clinical Nutrition,* 89(6), 1836-1845.

7. Engelmann, M.D., Sandström, B., & Michaelsen, K.F. (1998). Meat intake and iron status in late infancy: an intervention study. *Journal of Pediatric Gastroenterology and Nutrition,* 26(1), 26-33.

8. Rasmussen, K.M. (2001). Is there a causal relationship between iron deficiency or iron-deficiency anemia and weight at birth, length of gestation and perinatal mortality? *The Journal of Nutrition,* 131(2), 590S-603S.

9. www.clinicalcorrelations.org/?p=8405

10. Riordan, J., & Auerbach, K.G. (1999). Breast-related problems. *Breastfeeding and human lactation.* 2nd ed, 483-511. Jones and Bartlett Publishers.

11. Saavedra, J.M., Deming, D., Dattilo, A., & Reidy, K. (2013). Lessons from the feeding

infants and toddlers study in North America: what children eat, and implications for obesity prevention. *Annals of Nutrition and Metabolism*, 62(Suppl. 3), 27-36.

12. Reidy, K.C., Deming, D.M., Briefel, R.R., Fox, M.K., Saavedra, J.M., & Eldridge, A.L. (2017). Early development of dietary patterns: transitions in the contribution of food groups to total energy—Feeding Infants and Toddlers Study, 2008. *BMC Nutrition*, 3(1), 5.

13. Morley, R., Abbott, R., Fairweather-Tait, S., MacFadyen, U., Stephenson, T., & Lucas, A. (1999). Iron fortified follow-on formula from 9 to 18 months improves iron status but not development or growth: a randomised trial. *Archives of Disease in Childhood*, 81(3), 247-252.

14. Lozoff, B. (2011). Early iron deficiency has brain and behavior effects consistent with dopaminergic dysfunction. *The Journal of Nutrition*, 141(4), 740S-746S.

15. www.who.int/nutrition/publications/code_english.pdf

Chapter 5

1. ec.europa.eu/food/safety/labelling_nutrition/special_groups_food/children_en

2. www.who.int/publications/guidelines/nutrition/en/

3. Zand, N., Chowdhry, B.Z., Zotor, F.B., Wray, D.S., Amuna, P., & Pullen, F.S. (2011). Essential and trace elements content of commercial infant foods in the UK. *Food Chemistry*, 128(1), 123-128.

4. Cogswell, M.E., Gunn, J.P., Yuan, K., Park, S., & Merritt, R. (2015). Sodium and sugar in complementary infant and toddler foods sold in the United States. *Pediatrics*, peds-2014.

5. Melø, R., Gellein, K., Evje, L., & Syversen, T. (2008). Minerals and trace elements in commercial infant food. *Food and Chemical Toxicology*, 46(10), 3339-3342.

6. Di Giovinazzo, V. (2010). Towards an alternative paradigm of consumer behavior. (No.179).

7. Elliott, M.R., & Ravichandran, K.S. (2010). Clearance of apoptotic cells: implications in health and disease. *The Journal of Cell Biology*, 189(7), 1059-1070.

8. Hurley, K.M., & Black, M.M. (2010). Commercial baby food consumption and dietary variety in a statewide sample of infants receiving benefits from the special supplemental nutrition program for women, infants, and children. *Journal of the American Dietetic Association*, 110(10), 1537-1541.

9. García, A.L., Raza, S., Parrett, A., & Wright, C.M. (2013). Nutritional content of infant commercial weaning foods in the UK. *Archives of Disease in Childhood*, 98(10), 793-797.

10. Cogswell, M.E., Gunn, J.P., Yuan, K., Park, S., & Merritt, R. (2015). Sodium and sugar in complementary infant and toddler foods sold in the United States. *Pediatrics*, peds-2014.

11. Piccinelli, R., Pandelova, M., Le Donne, C., Ferrari, M., Schramm, K.W., & Leclercq, C. (2010). Design and preparation of market baskets of European Union commercial baby foods for the assessment of infant exposure to food chemicals and to their effects. *Food Additives and Contaminants*, 27(10), 1337-1351.

12. Ljung, K., Palm, B., Grandér, M., & Vahter, M. (2011). High concentrations of essential and toxic elements in infant formula and infant foods – a matter of concern. *Food Chemistry*, 127(3), 943-951.

13. Crawley, H. & Westland, S. (2017) *Baby Foods in the UK: A review of commercially produced jars and pouches of baby foods marketed in the UK*. First Steps Nutrition Trust.

14. Brown A, Lee, M.D. (2015) Early influences on child satiety-responsiveness: the role of weaning style. *Pediatric Obesity*. Feb 1;10(1):57-66.

15. Garcia, A.L., McLean, K., & Wright, C.M. (2015). Types of fruits and vegetables used in commercial baby foods and their contribution to sugar content. *Maternal & Child Nutrition*.

16. Foterek, K., Hilbig, A., Kersting, M., & Alexy, U. (2016). Age and time trends in the diet of young children: results of the DONALD study. *European Journal of Nutrition*, 55(2), 611-620.

17. Foterek, K., Hilbig, A., & Alexy, U. (2015). Associations between commercial complementary food consumption and fruit and vegetable intake in children. Results of the DONALD study. *Appetite*, 85, 84-90.

18. Randhawa, S., Kakuda, Y., Wong, C.L., & Yeung, D.L. (2012). Microbial safety, nutritive

value and residual pesticide levels are comparable among commercial, laboratory and homemade baby food samples — a pilot study. *Open Nutrition Journal*, 6, 89-96.

19. Smith-Spangler, C., Brandeau, M.L., Hunter, G.E., Bavinger, J.C., Pearson, M., Eschbach, P.J. ... & Olkin, I. (2012). Are organic foods safer or healthier than conventional alternatives?: a systematic review. *Annals of Internal Medicine*, 157(5), 348-366.

20. Dimitri, C., & Greene, C. (2000). Recent growth patterns in the US organic foods market. *Agriculture Information Bulletin*, 777.

21. www.who.int/nutrition/events/draft-inappropriate-promotion-infant-foods-en.pdf

22. Bentley, A. (2014). *Inventing Baby Food: Taste, Health, and the Industrialization of the American Diet* (Vol.51). Univ of California Press.

23. Hamilton, K., Daniels, L., Murray, N., White, K.M., & Walsh, A. (2012). Mothers' perceptions of introducing solids to their infant at six months of age: Identifying critical belief-based targets to promote adherence to current infant feeding guidelines. *Journal of Health Psychology*, 17(1), 121-131.

24. Hauck, Y.L., & Irurita, V.F. (2002). Constructing compatibility: managing breast-feeding and weaning from the mother's perspective. *Qualitative Health Research*, 12(7), 897-914.

25. Bui, M.D. Kaltcheva, V., Patino, A., & C. Leventhal, R. (2013). Front-of-package product labels: influences of varying nutritional food labels on parental decisions. *Journal of Product & Brand Management*, 22(5/6), 352-361.

26. Greiner, T., Latham, M.C. (1982) The influence of infant food advertising on infant feeding practices in St Vincent. *International Journal of Health Services*, 12(1):53-75

27. Berry, N.J., Jones, S.C., & Iverson, D. (2012). Toddler milk advertising in Australia: Infant formula advertising in disguise? *Australasian Marketing Journal*, 20(1), 24-27.

28. Berry, N.J., Jones, S., & Iverson, D. (2010). It's all formula to me: women's understandings of toddler milk ads. *Breastfeeding Review*, 18(1), 21.

29. Dickinson, R., Gunter, B., Matthews, J. & Cole, J. (2013) The Impact of Amended Controls on the Advertising of Infant Formula in the UK: Findings from a Before and after Study. *International Journal of Health Promotion and Education*, 51(1): 11-22.

30. NOP World for Department of Health. *Attitudes to feeding*. Report of survey findings. UK Crown, London 2005.

31. Frank, D.A., Wirtz, S.J., Sorensen, J.R. & Heeren, T. (1987) Commercial Discharge Packs and Breast-Feeding Counseling: Effects on Infant-Feeding Practices in a Randomized Trial. *Pediatrics* 80(6): 845-854.

Chapter 6

1. Rapley, G., Murkett, T. *Baby-led weaning: Helping your baby to love good food*. Random House; 2008

2. Wright, C.M., Cameron, K., Tsiaka, M., Parkinson, K.N. Is baby-led weaning feasible? When do babies first reach out for and eat finger foods? *Maternal & Child Nutrition*. 2011 Jan 1;7(1):27-33.

3. Rowan, H., Harris, C. (2012) Baby-led weaning and the family diet. A pilot study. *Appetite* 30;58(3):1046-9.

4. Brown, A., Lee, M. (2011) Maternal control of child feeding during the weaning period: differences between mothers following a baby-led or standard weaning approach. *Maternal and Child Health Journal*, 1;15(8):1265-71.

5. Cameron, S.L., Taylor, R.W., Heath, A.L. (2015) Development and pilot testing of Baby-Led Introduction to Solids – a version of Baby-Led Weaning modified to address concerns about iron deficiency, growth faltering and choking. *BMC Pediatrics*, 26;15(1):1.

6. Brown, A., Lee, M. (2013) An exploration of experiences of mothers following a baby-led weaning style: developmental readiness for complementary foods. *Maternal & Child Nutrition*, 1;9(2):233-43.

7. Cameron, S.L., Heath, A.L., Taylor, R.W. (2012) Healthcare professionals' and mothers' knowledge of, attitudes to and experiences with, Baby-Led Weaning: a content analysis study. *BMJ Open*, 1;2(6):e001542.

8.   Morison, B.J., Taylor, R.W., Haszard, J.J., Schramm, C.J., Erickson, L.W., Fangupo, L.J., Fleming, E.A., Luciano, A., Heath, A.L. (2016) How different are baby-led weaning and conventional complementary feeding? A cross-sectional study of infants aged 6–8 months. *BMJ Open*, 1;6(5):e010665.

9.   Brown, A., Lee, M.D. (2015) Early influences on child satiety-responsiveness: the role of weaning style. *Pediatric Obesity*, 1;10(1):57-66.

10. Townsend, E., Pitchford, N.J. (2012) Baby knows best? The impact of weaning style on food preferences and body mass index in early childhood in a case-controlled sample. *BMJ Open*, 1;2(1):e000298.

11. Fangupo, L.J., Heath, A.L., Williams, S.M., Williams, L.W., Morison, B.J., Fleming, E.A., Taylor, B.J., Wheeler, B.J., Taylor, R.W. (2016) A baby-led approach to eating solids and risk of choking. *Pediatrics* 19:e20160772.

12. Brown, A., Lee, M. (2013) Breastfeeding is associated with a maternal feeding style low in control from birth. *PLoS One*, Jan 30;8(1):e54229.

13. Brown, A., Lee, M. (2012) Breastfeeding during the first year promotes satiety responsiveness in children aged 18–24 months. *Pediatric Obesity*, Oct 1;7(5):382-90.

14. Wasser, H., Bentley, M., Borja, J., Goldman, B.D., Thompson, A., Slining, M. et al. (2011) Infants perceived as 'fussy' are more likely to receive complementary foods before 4 months. *Pediatrics* 127 (2), 229–237

15. Brown, A., Rowan, H. (2015). Maternal and infant factors associated with reasons for introducing solid foods. *Maternal & Child Nutrition*.

16. D'Andrea, E., Jenkins, K., Mathews, M., Roebothan, B. (2016) Baby-led Weaning: A Preliminary Investigation. *Canadian Journal of Dietetic Practice and Research*. Jan 15;77(2):72-7.

Chapter 7

1.   Black, M.M., & Aboud, F.E. (2011). Responsive feeding is embedded in a theoretical framework of responsive parenting. *The Journal of Nutrition*, 141(3), 490-494.

2.   Landry, S.H., Smith, K.E., & Swank, P.R. (2006). Responsive parenting: establishing early foundations for social, communication, and independent problem-solving skills. *Developmental Psychology*, 42(4), 627.

3.   World Health Organization. (2005). *Guiding principles for feeding non-breastfed children 6-24 months of age.*

4.   Blissett, J., Meyer, C., & Haycraft, E. (2006). Maternal and paternal controlling feeding practices with male and female children. *Appetite* 47, 212-219.

5.   Cooke, L.J., Wardle, J., Gibson, E.L., Sapochnik, M., Sheiham, A., & Lawson, M. (2004). Demographic, familial and trait predictors of fruit and vegetable consumption by pre-school children. *Public Health Nutrition*, 7(02), 295-302.

6.   Brown, J. & Ogden, J. (2004). Children's eating attitudes and behaviour: A study of the modelling and control theories of parental influence. *Health Education Research: Theory and Practice*, 19, 261-271.

7.   Birch, L.L., & Deysher, M. (1985). Conditioned and unconditioned caloric compensation: evidence for self-regulation of food by young children. *Learning and Motivation*, 16, 341-355.

8.   Fisher, J.O., & Birch, L.L. (1999b). Restricting access to palatable foods affects children's behavioural response, food selection and intake. *American Journal of Clinical Nutrition*, 69, 1264-1272.

9.   Liem, D.G., Mars, M., & De Graaf, C. (2004). Sweet preferences and sugar consumption of 4-and 5-year-old children: role of parents. *Appetite*, 43(3), 235-245.

10. Fisher, J.O., Birch, L., Smiciklas-Wright, H., & Piccano, M. (2000). Breastfeeding through the first year predicts maternal control in feeding and subsequent toddler energy intakes. *Journal of American Diet Association*, 100, 641-646.

11. Farrow, C., & Blissett, J. (2008).Controlling Feeding Practices: Cause or Consequence of early child weight? *Pediatrics*, 121, 1-6.

12. Faith, M.S., Scanlon, K.S., Birch, L.L., Francis, L.A., & Sherry, B. (2004). Parent-child feeding strategies and their relationships to child eating and weight status. *Obesity Research*, 12(11), 1711-1722.

13. Batsell, R., Brown, A., Ansfield, M., & Paschall, G. (2002). You will eat all of that! A retrospective analysis of forced consumption episodes. *Appetite*, 38, 211-219.

14. Galloway, A., Fiorito, L., Lee, Y. & Birch, L.L. (2005). Parental pressure, dietary patterns and weight status among girls who are picky eaters. *Journal of the American Dietetic Association*, 105, 541-8.

15. Birch, L.L., McPhee, L., Shoba, B., Steinberg, L., & Krehbiel, R. (1987). Clean up your plate: effects of child feeding on the conditioning of meal size. *Learning Motives*, 18, 301-317.

16. Benton, D. (2004). Role of parents in the determination of the food preferences of children and the development of obesity. *International Journal of Obesity*, 28, 858-869

17. Brann, L.S., & Skinner, J.D. (2005). More controlling child-feeding practices are found among parents of boys with an average body mass index compared with parents of boys with a high body mass index. *Journal of the American Dietetic Association*, 105, 1411-1416.

18. Farrow, C., & Blissett, J. (2008). Controlling Feeding Practices: Cause or Consequence of early child weight? *Pediatrics*, 121, 1-6.

19. Blissett, J., Haycraft, E., & Farrow, C. (2010). Inducing preschool children's emotional eating: relations with parental feeding practices. *The American Journal of Clinical Nutrition*, 92(2), 359-365.

20. Haycraft, E.L., & Blissett, J.M. (2008). Maternal and Parental controlling feeding practices: Reliability and Relationships with BMI. *Obesity*, 16, 1552-1558

21. Tiggemann, M. & Lowes, J. (2002). Predictors of maternal control over children's eating behaviour. *Appetite*, 39, 1-7.

22. Fisher, J.O., Rolls, B., & Birch, L.L. (2003). Children's bite size and intake of an entrée are greater with large portions than with age-appropriate or self-selected portions. *American Journal of Clinical Nutrition*, 77, 1164-70.

23. Jahnke, D.L., & Warschburger, P.A. (2008). Familial transmission of eating behaviours in preschool aged children. *Obesity*, 16/8, 1821-1825.

24. Dollberg, S., Lahav, S., Mimouni, F.B. (2001). A comparison of intakes of breastfed and bottle fed infants during the first two days of life. *Journal of the American College of Nutrition*, 20/3, 209-211.

25. Fomon, S.J., Owen, G.M., & Thomas, L.N. (1964). Milk or formula volume ingested by infants fed ad libitum. *American Journal of the Disorders of the Child*, 108, 601-612.

26. Agras, W.S., Kraemer, H.C., Berkowitz, R.I., Korner, A.F., & Hammer, L.D. (1987) Does a vigorous feeding style influence early development of adiposity. *Journal of Pediatrics* 110/5, 799-804.

27. Blissett, J., & Farrow, C. (2007). Predicting controlling feeding practices at one and two years. *International Journal of Obesity*, 31, 1520-1526.

28. Brown, A., & Lee, M. (2012). Breastfeeding during the first year promotes satiety responsiveness in children aged 18–24 months. *Pediatric Obesity*, 7(5), 382-390.

29. Li, R., Fein, S.B., & Grummer-Strawn, L.M. (2010). Do infants fed from bottles lack self-regulation of milk intake compared with directly breastfed infants?. *Pediatrics*, 125(6), e1386-e1393.

30. Kent, J.C., Mitoulas, L.R., Cregan, M.D. et al. (2006). Volume and frequency of breastfeedings and fat content of breast milk throughout the day. *Pediatrics*, 117, 387-395.

31. Konner, M., & Worthman, C. (1980). Nursing frequency, gonadal function, and birth spacing among !Kung hunter-gatherers. *Science*, 207(4432), 788-791.

32. Paul, K., Dittrichova, J. & Papousek, H. (1996). Infant feeding behaviour: development in patterns and motivation. *Developmental Psychobiology*, 29 (7) 563-576.

33. Richards, M.P.M., & Bernal, F. (1972). An observational study of mother-infant interaction. In N. Blurton Jones (Ed) *Ethological studies of child behaviour* (pp.175-197). Cambridge University Press.

34. Khan, S., Hepworth, A.R., Prime, D.K., Lai, C.T., Trengove, N.J., & Hartmann, P.E. (2013). Variation in fat, lactose, and protein composition in breast milk over 24 hours: associations with infant feeding patterns. *Journal of Human Lactation*, 29(1), 81-89.

35. Kent, J.C., Mitoulas, L.R., Cregan, M.D. et al. (2006). Volume and frequency of breastfeedings and fat content of breast milk throughout the day. *Pediatrics*, 117, 387-395.

36. Woolridge, M.W., Greasley, V., & Silpisornkosol, S. (1985). The initiation of lactation:

the effect of early versus delayed contact for suckling on milk intake in the first week post-partum. A study in Chiang Mai, Northern Thailand. *Early Human Development*, 12(3), 269-278.

37. Illingworth, R.S., Stone, D.H.G., Jowett, G.H., & Scott, J.F. (1952). Self-demand feeding in a maternity unit. *Lancet*, 1, 683-687.

38. de Carvalho, M., Robertson, S., Merkatz, R. & Klaus, M. (1982). Milk intake and frequency of feeding in breastfed infants. *Early Human Development*, 7, 155-163.

39. Woolridge, M.W., Greasley, V., & Silpisornkosol, S. (1985). The initiation of lactation: the effect of early versus delayed contact for suckling on milk intake in the first week post-partum. A study in Chiang Mai, Northern Thailand. *Early Human Development*, 12(3), 269-278.

40. Mennella, J.A., Jagnow, C.P., & Beauchamp, G.K. (2001). Prenatal and postnatal flavor learning by human infants. *Pediatrics*, 107(6), e88-e88.

41. ellynsatterinstitute.org/dor/divisionofresponsibilityinfeeding.php#sthash.vUQJNffU.dpuf

42. Farrow, C., & Blissett, J. (2006b). Does maternal control during feeding moderate early infant weight gain? *Pediatrics*, 118, 293-298.

43. Brown, A. (2014). Maternal restraint and external eating behaviour are associated with formula use or shorter breastfeeding duration. *Appetite*, 76, 30-35.

Chapter 8

1. Brown, A., & Rowan, H. (2016). Maternal and infant factors associated with reasons for introducing solid foods. *Maternal & Child Nutrition*, 12(3), 500-515.

2. McAndrew, F., Thompson, J., Fellows, L., Large, A., Speed, M., & Renfrew, M.J. (2015). *Infant Feeding Survey 2010*. Health and Social Care Information Centre.

3. Anders, T.F., Halpern, L.F., & Hua, J. (1992). Sleeping through the night: A developmental perspective. *Pediatrics*, 90, 554-560.

4. Macknin, M.L., Medendorp, S.V., & Maier, M.C. (1989). Infant sleep and bedtime cereal. *American Journal of Diseases of Children*, 143(9), 1066-1068.

5. Scher, A. (2001), Attachment and sleep: A study of night waking in 12-month-old infants. *Developmental Psychobiology*, 38, 274-285. doi:10.1002/dev.1020.

6. Ball, H.L. (2003), Breastfeeding, Bed-Sharing, and Infant Sleep. *Birth*, 30, 181–188. doi:10.1046/j.1523-536X.2003.00243.x.

7. O'Brien, L.M., & Gozal, D. (2004). Neurocognitive dysfunction and sleep in children: From human to rodent. *The Pediatric Clinics of North America*, 51, 187-202.

8. Price, A.M., Wake, M., Ukoumunne, O.C., & Hiscock, H. (2012). Five-year follow-up of harms and benefits of behavioral infant sleep intervention: randomized trial. *Pediatrics*, 130(4), 643-651.

9. Sellen, D.W. (2001). Weaning, complementary feeding, and maternal decision making in a rural east African pastoral population. *Journal of Human Lactation*, 17(3), 233-244.

10. Brown, A., & Harries, V. (2015). Infant sleep and night feeding patterns during later infancy: Association with breastfeeding frequency, daytime complementary food intake, and infant weight. *Breastfeeding Medicine*, 10(5), 246-252.

11. Doan, T., Gay, C.L., Kennedy, H.P., Newman, J., & Lee, K.A. (2014). Nighttime breastfeeding behavior is associated with more nocturnal sleep among first-time mothers at one month postpartum. *Journal of Clinical Sleep Medicine*, 10(3), 313-319.

12. McKenna, J.J., Ball, H.L., & Gettler, L.T. (2007). Mother-infant cosleeping, breastfeeding and sudden infant death syndrome: what biological anthropology has discovered about normal infant sleep and pediatric sleep medicine. *American Journal of Physical Anthropology*, 134(S45), 133-161.

13. Fildes, V.A. (1986). *Breasts, bottles and babies: a history of infant feeding*.

14. da Costa, T.H., Haisma, H., Wells, J.C., Mander, A.P., Whitehead, R.G., & Bluck, L.J. (2010). How much human milk do infants consume? Data from 12 countries using a standardized stable isotope methodology. *The Journal of Nutrition*, 140(12), 2227-2232.

15. Richardson, H.L., Walker, A.M., & Horne, R.S. (2010). Sleeping like a baby – does gender influence infant arousability?. *Sleep*, 33(8), 1055-1060.

16. Arnott, B., & Brown, A. (2013). An exploration of parenting behaviours and attitudes during early infancy: Association with maternal and infant characteristics. *Infant and Child Development*, 22(4), 349-361.

Index